The Beautiful Destruction of My Life

THE BEAUTIFUL *Destruction* OF MY LIFE

Finding hope in my Journey as a Wife, Mother, and Caregiver to a Disabled Veteran with Multiple System Atrophy

KIMBERLY S. BOHANNON

XULON ELITE

Xulon Press Elite
2301 Lucien Way #415
Maitland, FL 32751
407.339.4217
www.xulonpress.com

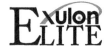

© 2023 by Kimberly S. Bohannon

All rights reserved solely by the author. The author guarantees all contents are original and do not infringe upon the legal rights of any other person or work. No part of this book may be reproduced in any form without the permission of the author. The views expressed in this book are not necessarily those of the publisher.

Due to the changing nature of the Internet, if there are any web addresses, links, or URLs included in this manuscript, these may have been altered and may no longer be accessible. The views and opinions shared in this book belong solely to the author and do not necessarily reflect those of the publisher. The publisher, therefore, disclaims responsibility for the views or opinions expressed within the work.

Unless otherwise indicated, Scripture quotations taken from the Holy Bible, New International Version (NIV). Copyright © 1973, 1978, 1984, 2011 by Biblica, Inc.™. Used by permission. All rights reserved.

Paperback ISBN-13: 978-1-66286-284-7
Ebook ISBN-13: 978-1-66286-285-4

Chapter 1

I'm lying in bed, wrapped in layers of blankets on a cold, snowy December Saturday morning; next to me lies my husband of twenty-one years. Though our bodies touch, the emotional space between us is miles apart.

My body is cold, not because the air is chilly, and I get easily cold. I'm cold because of the terrifying thoughts going through my mind. After years of marriage and two children, Steve and I are at a point where we are facing a divorce that will turn our lives topsy turvy. Tears stream down my face. *I don't feel either one of us thinks there is hope for a future together.*

The truth is harder than a lie. For a long time—years—I had lied to myself that our marriage was fine. It wasn't, and we both knew it. Now, we are tired of lying to each other.

I stare at the tiny snowflakes falling on the tall oak trees outside my window. As the snow is transforming the shape of the trees, so too would my life take on a different form. However, in that moment, I didn't know it wouldn't be from divorce but from a deeper commitment to our marriage that ultimately a tragedy would compel me to make.

My mind wanders to July 1987.

I grew up in Springfield Township, a suburb of Akron, Ohio. After graduating from high school in June 1986, I started college at the University of Akron in January 1987, hoping to get a BA in psychology.

I was the oldest of three girls. My middle sister Michelle is two years younger than me, and my youngest sister Melenie is seven years to the day younger than me. We had a unique bond growing up because I would refer to her as my twin born seven years apart.

Following my turbulent teen years, my mom and I weren't particularly close. I loved her, but we didn't have a strong, emotional connection. I used to attribute our lack of a strong bond to her life circumstances at the time. She was raising three girls with my dad working a lot, and they were struggling to pay the bills. Later I realized that our emotional distance also likely stemmed from her relationship with her mother, which was strained, and she lacked good role models and guidance. It was hard for her to show love because she had not received a lot of it growing up.

Despite this, my mom tried to give us the normal life she never had. She gave us homemade birthday parties and little treats at every single holiday. To this day, I hold a Valentine's Day party for my children, Jacob and Emily, just like my mom did for us.

In my free time, I went out with Mike, my high school sweetheart, or with Cheryl, a tall and lean pretty girl with short, dishwater blond hair and my best friend. Like me, she didn't participate in the typical high school drama over boys, and we connected immediately. Cheryl and I loved to shop, hang out in our cars and listen to music, and go for walks in a nearby park.

Chapter 1

By summer 1987, Cheryl and I, now nineteen, sought adventure. We decided to take our first official vacation—a trip to Orlando, Florida, to visit some friends we went to high school with, Don and Caroline. Don had joined the Navy after high school. He and Caroline had married, and they were living in an apartment near the Navy base in Orlando. This would be my first trip south of the Ohio border, the first time outside of the Buckeye State on my own. I was excited!

The night before we left, that excitement drained. My boyfriend Mike unexpectedly broke up with me, and excitement for the trip turned to sadness. Little did I know that sadness would dissipate in a flash as I soon would meet the love of my life.

Early the next morning, Cheryl and I hopped into her brand-new blue Chevy Cavalier, albeit without air conditioning or a radio, and hit the road for the eighteen-hour drive to Florida. I felt a strange hope for the future and must have had a premonition something was coming, something good.

We had packed her new car full of sandwiches, snacks, and gummi bears, as well as my boombox radio and extra batteries, though we could barely hear the radio with the windows down and the breeze blowing our hair. We didn't care. Our excitement about going to Florida fueled us for the long trip, and thoughts of Mike flew away with the cloudy Ohio skies.

We arrived in Orlando in the middle of a Saturday afternoon and went straight to Don and Caroline's apartment. They were the first friends I had ever visited that had their own apartment, as Cheryl and I both lived with our parents. Even Mike still lived with his parents.

Exhausted, we slept until dinner.

"I've got some friends in the Navy," Don said during dinner.

"I could set up a double date with them if you want."

Cheryl and I looked at each other, our faces beaming. "We'd love to," I said.

Steve and Jack were close friends of Don's from boot camp. Don called and arranged for them to stop by his apartment on their way home from the Naval Training Center in Orlando, where they both were attending Nuclear Field "A" School.

Cheryl and I were sitting in the living room on a cream-colored oversized sofa, waiting for the guys to arrive. They walked in the door. Wow! What handsome sailors. My mouth fell open, as did Cheryl's; it was instant chemistry for all four of us.

I was wearing green shorts and a matching light green tank top with tiny printed flowers and a pair of casual sandals; perfect for the Orlando heat and to show off my figure. To make a good first impression, I had curled my hair, reminiscent of the 1980's Farrah Fawcett, and put on a light foundtion, blush, and mascara. Never being too big on makeup, I put on enough to make it look like I wasn't trying too hard.

Cheryl fell for Jack, a good-looking guy from Wisconsin with glasses, very short wheat-colored hair, and a great sense of humor, and he fell for her as well. The same happened for Steve and me.

Chapter 1

Steve was from Athens, a small town in East Tennessee. Tall, a little over six feet, with short chestnut brown hair in a military haircut and wearing his white Navy summer uniform, he was handsome in a rugged kind of way and looked mature, older than me. Within minutes of meeting him, I knew we had something.

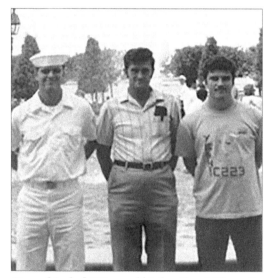

Steve, his dad Otto, and his brother Mike 1987

Exuding a quiet confidence, he strolled into Don's apartment, smoking a cigarette. My whole family smoked, but I had never dated anyone who smoked. Somehow his smoking appealed to me.

Our first conversation was brief. I was extremely nervous, and after the basic hellos, all I could think to say was, "How old are you?" How old was he? How embarrassing and such a dumb thing to ask. I felt like saying, "Well, la-di-da, la-di-da, la-la" as Annie Hall said to

Woody Allen in *Annie Hall* after an awkward moment right after meeting him. Oh well. La-di-da. I was nervous. Steve smiled and said, "I'm twenty."

After we got past the awkward conversation, Steve and I bantered about a bit, talking about the trip down from Ohio and about all of us going to high school together. Since it was my first trip to the Sunshine State, I asked Steve some basic questions about what it was like living in Florida and being in the Navy. I found it easy talking to him.

"Why don't you and Cheryl come over to my apartment tonight? We'll grill out," Steve said.

A grin spread from ear to ear. "We would love to," I blurted quickly, without asking Cheryl if that was okay. Cheryl's batting eyelashes and toothy smile confirmed that she was hooked on Jack and that was fine with her.

At 6:00 that night, the two of us waited in the apartment, butterflies in our stomachs. Finally, when Steve and Jack arrived to pick us up in Steve's late-model, light blue Chevy Camaro, we were beyond excited.

Jack hopped out. With a big smile on his face, he motioned me into the front seat. He opened the door for Cheryl to hop into the back seat, and then he sidled into the back seat on the other side. My handsome sailor had donned his navy suit for a pair of khaki shorts and a blue, plaid, button-down short-sleeved shirt. I wore a red jersey, knee-length summer dress. Nothing fancy, but it fit me just right.

Steve's apartment was twenty minutes away in Winter Haven. Thankfully, the windows were down, and it was loud outside, so I didn't have to come up with small talk.

Cheryl and Jack, meanwhile, were bantering away. Upon arriving to Steve's apartment complex, we went to the picnic tables at the outdoor pavilion so Steve could grill steaks for us. The weather in Orlando in July was hot, but to me, it felt like perfect weather.

"How do you want your steak cooked?" Steve asked. I had no idea. I never had a man cook for me before, let alone *a steak*. The only grilled food I had was a hamburger steak my dad grilled at home.

"Any way you want to," I said. For our entire marriage, Steve kidded me about my answer because he knows I like my steak more toward the well-done side while he likes his steaks medium-rare.

After dinner, Jack took Cheryl out for a drive and wound up back at Don and Caroline's apartment. Steve and I stayed at his apartment and talked for hours. I began to feel comfortable talking to him and told him about my life in Ohio, where I went to school, and where I worked.

We sat on his couch and talked for a long time. Warmth permeated my body, and I moved close to him. His head leaned into mine. Finally, he put his arm around me. I was nervous, but his arm around me felt so natural. I leaned my head into his neck. I felt at peace.

We were silent for a while. Finally, he leaned in and kissed me softly on the lips. This was the sweetest kiss I had ever had; the kind I had dreamed about from watching romantic movies. We kissed for a long time into the late hours of the night, with time eluding us.

Finally, Steve realized he had to take me back to our friend's apartment. By then, it was well past midnight.

Jack had left his own car at Steve's apartment, and then he and Steve rode over together to Don's to pick us up.

"What do you think?" Cheryl asked me, as I strolled in dreamy-eyed.

"I think I'm in love." I leaned my whole body against the doorway and rolled my eyes back. I was so young and naïve.

After our first date grilling steaks, Steve and I were inseparable, spending every free minute together in Orlando. We went out for pizza, cooked together, and even drove to Daytona Beach one night. Steve had to be at work at 7:00 a.m. each day at the base in Orlando, but that didn't stop us from staying up until at least 2:00 a.m. each night, talking about our hopes and dreams and falling for each other. At the end of the week, I knew I had met the man who would change my life.

Though we felt connected, our backgrounds couldn't have been more different.

He was from a small, rural town with farm animals in his backyard. I was from the city and saw farm animals only at a petting zoo for a school field trip. His family operated a cattle farm and drove trucks for a living. My father worked a desk job in the purchasing department of the electric company.

His family was strongly rooted in their Baptist faith. My family knew who God was but weren't devoted followers. His family went to church every time the doors were open while my family went once a year on Easter, with my excitement centered around the new Easter dress my mom had bought me. My dad used to joke that he

Chapter 1

went to church "St. Mattress," as having to sit through a sermon would put him immediately to sleep.

As the saying goes, opposites attract and meeting someone so different from me was exciting. Something about this quiet, terrifically good-looking guy in his white Navy uniform attracted me. While we didn't make long-term future plans, we did make plans to see each other the next month. We both sensed our lives were going to change.

There were problems, though. Shortly after meeting Steve, I learned he was married with a pending divorce. I had never known anyone who had been divorced.

His first wife was a couple of years younger than him. He told me they married when he joined the Navy and she was a senior in high school. She moved in with him after she graduated, but they lived together only for a week. Her parents drove to Florida and brought her back to Tennessee, and he did not believe she had any intentions of returning.

Looking back, I realize we should have waited for his divorce to finalize before starting a new relationship, but we were fools in love and felt like we knew more than anyone else.

Before I left, we didn't make any real plans. All Steve said was that he wanted me to come back, and he would visit me before my fall semester at the University of Akron started back.

How was I ever going to go back to Ohio?

Wearily and dreamingly, Cheryl and I took turns driving the eighteen hours back to Ohio without stopping to sleep. Pumped-up on Steve and Jack as if drugged, we talked non-stop about them the whole trip home.

Excitedly, we made plans to return to Orlando as soon as possible. One month later, we were both on a flight to Orlando for a second week.

When I got off the plane in Orlando, Steve was waiting for me. He looked more handsome than I remembered. My eyes lit up, and I ran into his arms. He enveloped me, and I melted into him, my heart pounding away. It was the happiest moment in my nineteen years.

He kissed me, sweetly and tenderly. I vowed to never let go of this man. Hands locked, we walked back to his car. I stayed at Steve's apartment and Cheryl and Jack stayed at Don and Caroline's apartment.

Again, Steve and I spent every possible minute together and fell hard for each other. We took a weekend trip to Cocoa Beach and talked for hours every night until the middle of the night. He borrowed Don's motorcycle and took me riding several nights.

We spent our time like a normal couple, going to the grocery store and cleaning the apartment. So much about him was new and exciting. On my eyes were rose-colored glasses and nothing short of surgery would remove them, as this man could do or say no wrong.

During our week together, I tried to impress him with my domestic skills by cooking a meal for him. However, this was not my best idea.

Steve's mom is one of the best Southern cooks I've ever met. Everything she made was from scratch and included a laundry list of ingredients not found in the average kitchen. The meal generally simmered for many hours to achieve the delightful aroma that exuded from her kitchen.

Chapter 1

Having grown up on her home-cooking, Steve, too, loved to cook. I learned my cooking from Home Economics class in high school. "Home Ec" included several ways of making canned biscuits into pizza and some basic soup recipes. Cooking was a skill I rarely practiced at home unless putting a frozen dinner in the oven counts.

Of course, Steve's family rarely, if ever, ate packaged meals. Almost everything was created from a recipe and not from the frozen food section. Nevertheless, that night I did somehow manage to make a basic beef roast with potatoes and carrots that I didn't mess up too badly.

At the end of the week, Steve and Jack drove us to the airport. Steve and I held hands, waiting for my flight. We hardly said a word, devastated at having to part from one other. Steve walked me toward the gate. Before I entered the tunnel to depart, he pulled me close and, with tears in his eyes, said, "I am going to marry you someday."

Tears streamed down my eyes, and I tightly hugged him. Wrenching apart from each other was torture. Though we had spent only a couple of weeks together, we were crazy about each other. He was everything I wanted: tall, handsome, and intelligent; riding motorcycles and had a cool, light blue Chevy Camaro; a man serving his country who knew what he wanted to do with his life.

Tears flowed the whole way back to Ohio. Self-consciously, I wiped my eyes and turned away from the flight attendant, worried she would ask me if I was okay. Cheryl was crying too. She and Jack were headed down exactly the same path, and it was clear they were falling for each other. They ended up marrying the same year that Steve and I married and are still married to this day. I see them every time I visit Ohio, and we all stayed close over the years.

Steve and I decided we would figure out a way to be together. Six months after meeting, he was transferred to the USS John F. Kennedy, an aircraft carrier stationed in Norfolk, Virginia. He worked in the bowels of the ship in the electrical motor rewind shop. His days were long and involved, using strong chemicals to strip the copper wiring from motors and rewinding them.

As soon as my last semester at the University of Akron was finished, I packed what few items I owned and moved to Norfolk to live with Steve, intending on going to college in Norfolk.

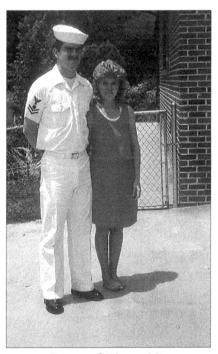

Steve and Kim 1988

Chapter 1

I told my parents I needed to live with Steve to see if I wanted to marry him. Though my parents didn't like me moving away, they said little about us moving in together. My parents were fairly liberal with me, but they didn't express a strong opinion of Steve. All they said was, "You should wait until he is actually divorced." His divorce was final in December, and I moved in with him in January.

I always felt fortunate that I had a good relationship with my parents growing up. My mom and I had typical teenage struggles. I was stubborn and thought I knew everything and generally questioned my mom on anything she told me. My dad was easygoing, and we got along great.

My dad spent most of his time working at the Ohio Edison Electric Company or tinkering in the garage on a small engine repair business he owned. I liked to spend time with my dad on weekends, going to old car shows, county fairs, and tractor pulls. Often, my dad and I would hop in the car and go to the A&W drive-in for frothy root beers and delicious onion rings. While my parents may not have lavished me with "I love you" daily, I always felt loved and secure.

Steve's parents were conservative, so he never told them we moved in together; rather, he lived on the ship and me in a nearby apartment.

Steve and I had few conversations about getting married. We both just assumed we would someday.

A few months after I moved to Norfolk, Steve found out he would be deployed for six months at sea on a Mediterranean Cruise; this was not the news I wanted to hear. I hardly knew anyone in Norfolk and would now be alone in a strange town for at least six months. Fortunately, I had started working as a bank teller, my first full-time job, and I loved it.

About a month before Steve was to deploy, we decided to get married. There was no fancy proposal. He didn't get down on one knee and tell me he couldn't live without me. He just said, "When can you take a day off of work and get married?" I didn't care that it wasn't a fancy proposal. I just wanted to be married to him.

The week before we married, we told my parents and grandparents. My parents didn't say much, though my mom did say, "I hope this is what you want." Not exactly the congratulations I was looking for, but looking back now, I understand why she said this.

My grandmother Dorothy had the most to say about me getting married. "Are you pregnant? Is that why you are getting married?"

"Grandma, of course not. Why would you ask that? I love him and want to marry him before he deploys out to sea for six months." I was baffled by her question. Didn't she think people got married just because they were crazy in love? Many years after my grandmother died, I learned that she and my grandfather had eloped because she was pregnant with a son who was later stillborn.

We didn't tell Steve's parents we were getting married. He had only been officially divorced for seven months at this point, and we felt they might not be supportive. Looking back, I now understand why.

One year after we initially met , on Thursday, July 7, 1988, a hot afternoon in Norfolk, in my blue Chevy S10, without air conditioning or a radio, we drove around

Chapter 1

downtown searching the courthouse for the justice of the peace to marry us. Well before cellphones and GPS, we almost missed our own wedding because we couldn't find the courthouse. After my first attempt at a government-looking building that turned out to be the Social Security Administration, we finally found the Norfolk Circuit Court Clerk's Office. There were no witnesses: just Steve, the judge, and me.

Steve wore a blue-striped polo shirt and nice gray slacks. He had such good taste, and it was wonderful to see him dressed up. I wore a knee-length, short-sleeved pink dress with a lacy lapel and little flowers all over it. This dress had seen its share of wedding vows. I had worn it a couple of years before to Don and Caroline's wedding, and more recently when my grandparents renewed their vows for their fiftieth wedding anniversary. It was the nicest dress I owned.

We couldn't afford to take a honeymoon, but thankfully, my grandmother mailed us a check for fifty dollars. She had eloped when she was about our age and understood some of what we were facing. It was the only wedding present we received and, thanks to her wedding present, we enjoyed a nice dinner that night at a fancy restaurant, where we ate steak by candlelight. Though in love and happy, we had obstacles to overcome.

Going through a divorce had left a part of Steve damaged and always somewhat emotionally detached. I was too young and naïve to see that part of his quietness and ruggedness was actually the emotional walls he put around himself to protect him from being vulnerable again. He didn't want a divorce from his first wife and wanted things to work out between them. He told me he felt he had failed when he got a divorce. He carried this perceived failure throughout our marriage, worried he would fail again, and now today, almost twenty years later in our marriage, as Steve and I are contemplating a divorce, he would face it again.

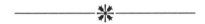

As I am getting out of my mind and pondering the meaning of the decision I'm about to make, I run my fingers through my long, blond hair, trying to straighten out the tousled mess. My hair desperately needs the roots touched-up. Who has the time? The farm and kids eat up all time.

How did we get here? My head's spinning. We spent a lifetime making selfish, immature choices. I think about how I put my wants in front of Steve's happiness. I don't think we've been on an actual date alone in ten years!

I think about how I enjoy spending time with the kids more than time with Steve and think he feels the same. He laughs and jokes with the kids but rarely with me. What happened? We had been so happy when we first got married, and I was a handsome sailor's wife. How did things slide? I think back on those early days of our marriage.

For eight months after we married, Steve was deployed in Operation Desert Storm and at sea on the aircraft carrier USS John F. Kennedy (CV-67). After nearly four years at Norfolk, he was transferred to USNS Roosevelt Roads in Ceiba, Puerto Rico.

Chapter 1

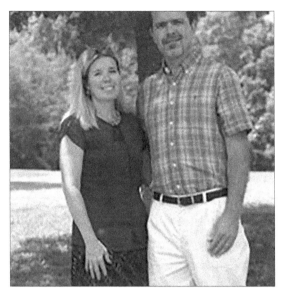

Kim and Steve

We loved Puerto Rico and quickly absorbed the culture and beautiful weather. We lived in military family housing on the base. I got a job at the Navy Federal Credit Union on base, and we quickly met a group of other military families. Brenda, a pretty, energetic, dark-haired woman with a sweet, easygoing personality, and her smart and handsome husband Russ were good friends. Very handy, he liked to do small home improvement projects, often repurposing old children's toys left out for recycling into plant stands for Brenda. Closer in age to my parents than to us, they looked out for everyone in our group.

Kraig, a young, single blond-haired guy from Connecticut, Debbie, short, petite, funny, and easy to talk to, and her husband Alan all became our family on the Navy base. Debbie was from Texas and on active duty in the Navy, introduced to us through another friend. Russ and Kraig were both on active duty in the Navy with Steve, and they all worked together at the security detachment. This group became our makeshift family, and we closely connected, eating meals together, celebrating holidays and birthdays, and becoming each other's support system.

In 1995, Steve was transferred to the Naval Reserve Center in Greensboro, North Carolina, and after fourteen years in the Navy as an electrician's mate, this would become his last duty station in the Navy. We spent five years in North Carolina and, in 2000, after having our son Jacob in 1996 while we were still in North Carolina, and our daughter Emily almost two years later, he decided it was time to leave the Navy and return to his hometown to be closer to family members..

Though we both had full-time jobs when Jacob and Emily were born, we lived paycheck to paycheck. We paid our bills and were never behind, but neither were we ever ahead. We never had money in savings, always carried a balance on our credit card that we couldn't pay off and lived one appliance breakdown away from more trouble.

Hoping to improve our situation, we made plans to move back to Steve's hometown of Athens, a farm town in eastern Tennessee. Steve immediately received a job offer as purchasing manager for a medical imaging company. I was able to continue a job I had at a credit union trade association, by working mostly from home.

Living in Athens was a great move for our family, as we finally had a family support system to lean on. As a military family, one of the biggest struggles had been not having family or close friends to turn to for help, even for little things like running an errand or childcare. Still, I missed having my own family nearby.

At first, moving back to Tennessee to manage the family farm had sounded romantic. Steve's parents owned nearly 300 acres among multiple farms. His dad had recently retired from truck driving but was not in good enough health to farm full time. Steve made it his mission to sustain the family farm, along with working his job at the medical imaging company an hour away in Knoxville.

Farming had been a foreign concept to me; we didn't even have a garden in suburban Ohio. So, out of necessity, Steve taught me how to help manage the farm. I could drive the tractor, rake hay, even helped load cows, and once helped our nanny birth a set of twin goats. Still, the farm was and always would be more of Steve's life dream, not mine.

I dreaded the time and money doing so would involve. Despite the notion of hobby farming, it's a full-time job and a very expensive hobby. In the summer, Steve mowed and baled hay from early in the morning until evening on weekends and days off. In the winter, he fed the cows hay several nights each week after work, and in the fall, we usually spent every Saturday fixing the fence and doing maintenance on the barn and gates. His dad had been unable to keep up the maintenance on the farm in previous years due to his failing health, and it would take quite a financial investment to get the farm in shape again.

Steve's dream had been to make the farm self-sustainable and his full-time job. To achieve this, he would have to spend every waking moment farming when he wasn't at his full time job.

He did. We spent thousands of dollars each year purchasing cattle to build up the herd and purchasing a hay baler, tractor, gooseneck trailer, mowing machine, hay rake, feed, and replacing miles of fencing and gates. I knew we had to invest money to make money, but this farm seemed an endless pit of expenses and drained our resources.

With so much money going into improving and building up the farm, we didn't have extra to put into a nice house. We had to live in a patched-together house on a small lot about five miles from Steve's parents' farm. We had bought the house sight unseen for a great price when we were moving back from North Carolina. We thought we could put a little money into fixing it up and make it work, but we were quite mistaken.

The first year we lived in the house, we were constantly spending money to make this fixer-upper livable. Our first mistake as naïve fixer-uppers was not checking the structural integrity of the house. The foundation wasn't solid, the floors were at varying degrees of level, and we didn't have a heating and air system for the first couple of years. We relied on a wood stove in the wintertime to heat the whole house and sweltered in the East Tennessee summers without A/C. We were living in the early nineteenth century!

I envied family and friends who had much nicer houses and took vacations and went to the lake on Saturdays while our vacations consisted of taking the kids to visit my family in Ohio. On Saturdays, Steve was out the door by 7:00 a.m., rarely coming home before dark.

I loved the farm but regretted how it consumed Steve's time and interests. Feeding and managing the cows and driving the truck to pick up hay took priority over our dreams. We had talked about building a house together someday, but because of time and money poured into this farm, that seemed remote.

The farm became a mistress in our marriage, and I resented it. It was the farm, along with both of us committed to our jobs: Steve as purchasing manager for a medical imaging company and me as the vice president for a credit union trade association. While we both were committed to doing things with Jacob and Emily, we had little time for each other. On top of it, we were each traveling for work, where Steve was gone one week, and I would take off the next.

I looked forward to my week away as an escape from the unhappiness that loomed over us like a dark storm cloud. I felt paralyzed and wanted to break free from this suffocation of unhappiness. I wanted to know what it was like to love in some deep and perfect way.

Now, I lie in bed, dreading the inevitable talk we both have avoided for too long.

Steve comes in the room and I bolt up. We look at each other, and I finally say the words, "I think we should separate. It is clear we are both unhappy." I can't say the word "divorce," but we both know what this means. We have never considered separating before. How did we get to this point?

Steve and I have never been good about communicating what we are thinking. The oldest child in our families, we are used to getting our way. I have never considered putting his needs over my own because I am my own person. Now I'm not so sure who I am anymore.

He is more stubborn than I am, and during an argument, I usually give in to keep the peace. Instead of talking to him about what I want and how we can work together, I shut down emotionally and resent him.

I know he loves me, but I never feel important in his life. I feel like loving me is a requirement because we are married, but enjoying my company is optional. *Does he want me more than the farm? Does he need me more than the farm? Can I be replaced if I refuse to go along with his plans?* I'm sure he has the same insecurities about me, as he, too, likely wonders if he is indispensable in *my* life.

The conversation about the state of our marriage between us drags, feeling like it can go on for hours. We don't argue, cry, or yell and threaten as I am expecting. This is how we normally deal with our problems. Rather, we have a sobering conversation. Why couldn't we have talked like this before?

Suddenly, Steve looks at his watch, and we know we will have to pick up the conversation later. It is Saturday morning, and that means putting out hay to feed the herd of cows. In addition to Steve's full-time job and my own, we manage more than fifty cows he keeps on his parents' farm.

Chapter 1

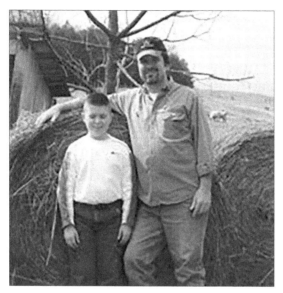

Jacob and Steve on the farm

Steve leaves for the farm, and I do my usual Saturday cleaning and cooking. All day I pray and make peace with whatever decision we come to.

I dread Steve returning home this afternoon, but we *have* to come to a decision. I shudder. How will we tell Jacob, our thirteen-year-old, or Emily, our eleven-year-old, that their parents are going to separate? They, too, are struggling with the throes of beginning adolescence. Neither one needs further change to disrupt their lives and equanimity.

When Steve walks in the door later in the day, something strange happens. He appears joyful despite what we are facing. How can his attitude have changed so drastically from this morning? Maybe he realizes how good life will be without me?

He comes in the kitchen and sits down at one of the wooden barstools at the kitchen counter. I am at the stove cooking. For some reason, I decide today is the day to spend some time in the kitchen. I feel like I might soon lose this opportunity to have a meal with our family together; it is almost as if I am fixing our last supper. I prepare a turkey, homemade creamed potatoes, green beans, and all the fixings.

"I've had a life-transforming experience. It's given me a change of heart," Steve says.

"What happened?" I ask.

He proceeds to tell me. While driving in his big, white, diesel, four-door F250 truck that we can barely afford, he was listening to a preacher on the radio. He tells me he doesn't even remember turning this station on when he got in the truck earlier. However, the radio preacher said something as though talking to Steve alone, not another soul listening. He says, "There is someone out there facing a difficult decision. I want you to know if God can bring you to it—God will bring you through it."

"That's the answer I've been searching for," Steve says to me.

I am confused. Why would God allow us the grace to repair our marriage and build it even stronger? I don't understand. How will it be possible to love Steve in a way I have never loved him in our twenty-one years of marriage?

It wasn't until later that I learned God had a specific plan and purpose to restore our marriage. The words the radio preacher spoke would come to symbolize our journey together over the next six years, as we would soon

Chapter 1

face the most difficult trial our marriage, *any* marriage, could ever endure.

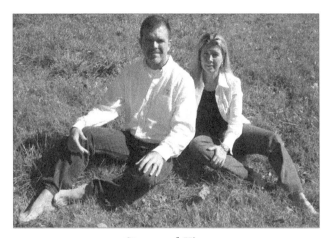

Steve and Kim

Chapter 2

*I*n 2005, Steve had started seeing a urologist. He was experiencing bouts of urinary incontinence that seemed unusual and began when he was only thirty-five. We were also rarely intimate anymore; I thought it was just part of his disdain for our marriage. I never realized there was an actual medical problem occurring or connected the two different medical problems he was experiencing together. To me, they were just part of our poor marriage at the time, and we all faced at some point getting older. I soon learned the impotence bothered him tremendously, and he had started taking Viagra without telling me in hopes of improvement.

The urinary incontinence increased, and in 2007, he received a diagnosis of tethered cord syndrome, a rare disease that typically presents with multiple neurological symptoms, including lower extremity pain, backache, lower extremity muscle weakness, and bowel/bladder disturbances.

It made sense to the doctors and us. He had a lot of back problems over the years and had surgery for it. The detethering procedure involved separating the spinal cord from the tissue of the spinal column. In nearly every case, this surgery permanently alleviates TCS symptoms, but in Steve, there was no change.

At first, Steve's symptoms seemed to improve. However, about eight weeks into his recovery, all of his symptoms returned. After a year of no improvement, his doctor recommended a second more invasive surgery for his tethered cord. Again, Steve endured a surgical procedure for it, but within eight weeks of leaving the hospital after surgery, his urinary incontinence started again. Could the doctors have been wrong? We didn't know what to think.

In 2008, he started having night sweats and constipation. The constipation became severe. He tried every over-the-counter laxative and lots of old remedies passed down from family members and well-meaning friends, but no remedy seemed to improve it. He also started to experience muscle weakness on his right side. He would tell me that his right leg felt like dead weight, and his right arm would tremor when he was stressed.

He could still ride his motorcycle, but I noticed that his leg bothered him. He had to stop and rest more often when riding, and he would drag his leg slightly when walking. He also had trouble maintaining body temperature. For years, Steve and I struggled with his temperature issues because he was always hot, and I was always cold. However, for the first time in our lives, we were both cold.

Chapter 2

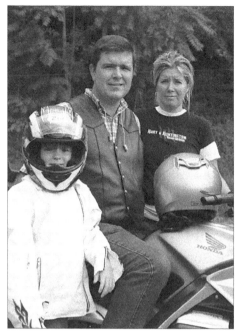

Emily, Steve, and Kim

By 2009, life, as we knew it, had irrevocably changed. Steve could no longer lift his right leg. Unable to manage riding his Honda-touring motorcycle, he sold it, which killed him to do so as we both loved riding the motorcycle. Riding on the back, my arms around him as he drove, was the closest we came to a connection.

In August, Steve picked me up from work one day with the kids. A handicap parking placard hung from the rearview mirror. He had never even told me he was going to apply for one. Though I tried my best to hide it from him, I was embarrassed. I didn't think he needed one.

I had been in denial. Now, the reality of the handicap parking sign forced me to really look at him and pay attention to how he walked with difficulty. Before this point, I had noticed some slow movement, but I guess I was completely blinded to what was happening. His gait was very slow and deliberate, almost as if his right leg didn't want to keep up with his left leg.

Watching my forty-two-year-old husband hardly able to walk was a pivotal moment. Something was wrong, not just a lot of odd symptoms. I said nothing and retreated into denial, unable to face what was in front of my nose.

By 2010, Steve's health continued to decline. Along with urinary incontinence, he had trouble maintaining his blood pressure and would have bouts of unexplained low blood pressure, along with severe muscle weakness, a wet sensation in his legs, headaches, and short-term memory loss. For instance, he would ask me where he had placed his keys. It was completely normal for me to lose my keys on a regular basis, but Steve never forgot where he placed his keys.

Several nights he had awakened me in the middle of the night to change the sheets because he had wet the bed. He never even knew it was happening. One time at work, he had to leave early and go home because he had wet himself at work and didn't even realize it. Thankfully, he had dark jeans on that day, and no one noticed.

Steve tried to hide as many symptoms from me as possible. He was struggling with the pain from headaches but didn't want me to know, taking handfuls of ibuprofens each day, and I didn't even realize it. He didn't tell me his muscles were achy and weak. Was he trying to protect me, his pride, or both? I wasn't sure.

He made regular visits to the Veterans Administration medical clinics in Tennessee in search of a diagnosis.

Since he had a full-time job with health insurance, he also met with every specialist recommended in the state in search of a diagnosis. I went with him to several of the appointments.

Unfortunately, every doctor uttered the same phrase "You have a very unusual case."

Finally, in early 2010, Steve was referred to a neurologist in Knoxville, who diagnosed him with Parkinson's disease.

Parkinson's is a disorder of the central nervous system that leads to shaking, stiffness, and difficulty with walking, balance, and coordination. Symptoms usually begin gradually and get worse over time. As the disease progresses, people may have difficulty walking, talking, and may have incontinence and constipation because the messages from the brain to the bladder or bowel get disrupted.

Steve seemed to have all these symptoms, but at forty-three, he seemed young for a Parkinson's diagnosis. The average age of someone diagnosed with Parkinson's disease is fifty-six. Only 4 percent of Parkinson's patients are diagnosed before the age of fifty.

Parkinson's was both a devastating diagnosis and a relief to us. We felt we finally knew what we were dealing with and could develop a treatment plan. I remember talking to my mom on the phone, telling her Steve was diagnosed with Parkinson's. Even as I said the words out loud for some reason, I didn't believe it myself.

Most importantly, a few months before Steve's Parkinson's diagnosis, we committed to rebuild our marriage. Deep in my soul, I felt if there was a glimmer of hope left, I didn't want to throw away twenty-two years of marriage. I didn't want to give up.

Many years back, after Steve and I got married, I had accepted Christ as my personal Savior but never committed myself to God. I was actively attending church, but I wasn't where I needed to be with my faith. Now, after Steve's diagnosis, I recommitted my life to God, becoming hungry for reading and absorbing my Bible and working to strengthen my faith and marriage.

We went to a Christian counselor to learn how to communicate and what God's plan was for our marriage. Our counselor was an older man named Gary with curly gray hair and a very jovial way of communicating. He loved to talk about his family, and in some sessions, I felt like we talked about his family as much as saving our own.

We went to see him every week for several months. It was the best investment we could have made in our marriage, as Gary pushed us to talk about our problems. Before counseling, Steve and I generally avoided doing so. If we were mad at each other, we waited for it to go away and never discussed how it made us feel. We just swept our problems under the rug, and there was a lot under it. Thankfully, Steve and I emerged from counseling with a new understanding of each other and a renewed appreciation for how God wanted us to treat each other. Most importantly, we set our differences aside and fell into a much deeper love with each other.

My commitment was now to care for Steve, and I would do all in my power to do so. The first thing I did was change jobs.

Chapter 2

Steve and I both had good jobs and traveled a lot for work. I generally went back and forth between our home in Tennessee and my company headquarters in North Carolina at least one week a month. As a purchasing manager, Steve often traveled to different plants to audit them, which took him all over the country and sometimes overseas, including trips to Mexico, Canada, and Germany.

We had tried to alternate our schedules so that one of us was always home at night. During the day, the kids were in school, and we had afterschool care. When Steve first began to get sick and problems like walking got worse, God led me to look for a new job closer to Knoxville, Tennessee, where I wouldn't have to travel back and forth from the company's headquarters in Greensboro, North Carolina.

Steve's employer had been very understanding, and he had already stopped traveling. I think his boss and coworkers could see how much he was physically starting to struggle to walk from his car to his office area each day. His movement was slowed to the point that he really could have used a cane to keep him steady. He told his boss he could not travel temporarily, which was honest since he didn't know exactly what this was or how long it would last. However, he continued to drive to the office every day to keep working. They provided him a small office near the elevator so he wouldn't have to take the stairs and even provided him a designated parking spot near the elevator.

The move for me was difficult. I loved my job and had no interest in leaving it, and Steve knew it. I regularly prayed, trying to figure out how I could keep my current job without moving back to North Carolina or continuing to travel. An answer came quickly.

An opportunity opened closer to home that did not involve overnight travel. I would be working every day from a single office. It was less pay, less seniority, and I would have to commute an hour to work each day, but I could still do what I loved as a compliance officer in a credit union. God had a beautiful plan at work here for me to leave my job in North Carolina and gain a whole new family at my new job at the credit union in Knoxville. I could never have imagined that God would take away a good job to provide me a much better job, but that's what happened.

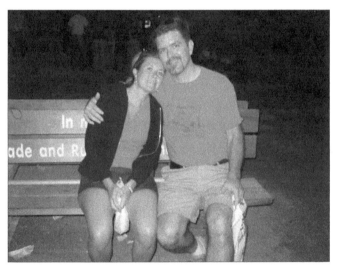

Kim and Steve

Chapter 3

*I*nitially, Steve had accepted the diagnosis of Parkinson's disease and for the first six months, took every medication known to help with Parkinson's: Carbidopa-levodopa, dopamine agonists, MAO B inhibitors, Catechol O-methyltransferase (COMT) inhibitors, anticholinergics, amantadine, and so on. None made a dent in Steve's symptoms. The doctors were baffled and unable to explain why the medicines weren't helping him. Finally, they began to question the diagnosis. Maybe it wasn't Parkinson's, but what was it?

I had been at my new job for about six months when, finally, Steve's primary care doctor had agreed to request that the Mayo Clinic, a world-class clinic in Rochester, Minnesota, specializing in rare diseases, evaluate his case. It took months of waiting before the Mayo Clinic agreed to see Steve and review his medical case.

This was both a blessing and a problem. The visit to the clinic in Minnesota would mean at least a 2,000-mile round trip. They told us to plan to stay for up to two weeks while seeing doctors at the clinic.

We considered flying to the Mayo Clinic but couldn't afford it. The visit to the Mayo Clinic did not have a definite set of appointments. They would set up some initial diagnostic appointments and then the doctors at those appointments would determine additional appointments. Round-trip plane tickets and fees associated with changing the tickets and a rental car were too steep for our finances.

The best scenario was to drive to Minnesota. Despite Steve struggling to walk, he wanted to attempt driving. He was trying to hold onto any opportunity to be the provider in our marriage and be in control of his own life.

He also loved driving. Throughout our marriage, I rarely drove when we were together. It wasn't that I was a bad driver; I just deferred to Steve because he loved to drive and travel. Before we had kids, Steve even asked me to consider a career change from my credit union job.

"Hey, let's go out on the road and see the country while we earn a living," Steve mentioned.

"Are you crazy? I hate the idea of being cooped up in a truck twenty-four hours a day," I stated.

"Yeah but think about everything we will get to see and we can be home every weekend."

"No! I will not even entertain the thought in my brain. Few things would make me unhappier than being a long-distance truck driver! I like prolonged driving as much as I like a root canal, and I'm quite certain I have zero ability to park a big truck, let alone back one up with a trailer."

He laughed, and I huffed.

"Do you remember the time I tried to back up the small, eight-foot trailer we have?" I asked. "I was so turned around I had to stop and unhook and drag the trailer by hand to the place it was supposed to be because I was so frustrated. Thankfully for you, it was not loaded."

On the way to the Mayo Clinic, we planned on taking turns driving and splitting the trip into almost three days each way to allow Steve time to rest.

That ended up meaning at least two weeks off work. At that point, I had only two days' vacation time built up. I would miss out on pay and, as a new employee, I was afraid to ask for two weeks' time off work in my first six months of employment. I wasn't sure if my employer would even grant the request. Even if they did, I would be without pay for approximately two weeks, and medical bills were mounting, but we couldn't turn down the appointment, as it was our best and, perhaps only, hope of a diagnosis for Steve.

God's plan was at work and gave me the courage to approach my company with my dilemma. Embracing me like a valuable part of their family, the credit union, my new company, generously allowed me the time off I needed to go with Steve. In addition to allowing me time off work, they also allowed me to apply for paid time off through their employee vacation donation bank.

Each year, long-term employees with excess vacation time may donate some of their vacation time to a bank for other employees in need. Throughout the whole ordeal of our journey of finding out what was causing Steve's illness, this fantastic credit union family provided a loving and caring environment. To this day, I am eternally grateful for the caring staff that work there.

The CEO and senior leadership team regularly took time to stop by my office and ask me how Steve was doing, and if there was anything they could do for our family. It meant a lot to me to know the leadership of our credit union truly cared about the families of their employees.

This trip would be a turning point for Steve's independence. On our first visit to the clinic, he could still drive much of the 1,000-mile trip there. However, that would be the last time he could drive.

He had somehow continued working between regular doctor visits as well, but now we were faced with a hard reality. He was severely constipated, spending about two hours per day in the bathroom. We tried every over-the-counter remedy, every remedy a family member had ever heard of, and daily enemas, but nothing worked. He had to stop almost every hour to urinate and even then, sometimes couldn't go. He would have a sudden urge to go and then nothing would come out. We both knew he could no longer work. Even walking unassisted was increasingly harder for him.

Steve's independence and mine as well took another hit. The two-week 2,000-mile round trip to Mayo Clinic would be a financial strain. Steve and I had been independent and wouldn't ask our families for help, but later, God would forcefully break us from that bad habit of pride.

Unexpectedly, Steve's coworker Kim rallied all his friends together and took care of us. Kim, a kindhearted close friend of Steve's at work. She and Steve had developed a close bond. They shared a love of cookbooks and recipes, with Steve like a brother to her to whom she looked to for advice.

Chapter 3

One day at work, Kim delivered a box to me from Steve's coworkers. I waited until I got home so we could open it together.

What a shock. We both burst into tears. Inside the cardboard box were cards by many of his coworkers, including notes of encouragement for the impending doctor visits, snacks, reading material, and other goodies for the trip.

That wasn't all. Inside the box were gift cards to purchase gas for the trip and fast food, along with cash for hotel rooms to make the trip. Their generosity made that trip possible.

Finally, after a couple of years and a lot of "you have a very unusual case" responses from every "ologist," we were going to have the opportunity to meet with doctors at this clinic. I was certain they would know the name of this mystery illness we were dealing with.

Prior to this appointment, I had watched every episode of "Mystery Diagnosis" on TV. I was convinced one day, I would see someone with similar symptoms as Steve, and we would figure this out. Unbeknownst to me, Steve already had his suspicions on what the disease was.

An expert at research and working in the medical field, Steve had, without telling me, been researching diseases with his symptoms for the last couple of years and had read every medical journal and research paper he could get his hands on and began developing a suspicion on what it was.

He had kept me in the dark about his discovery, though. The only thing he told me was that from his research, he knew his symptoms were serious. Cancer came to my mind, but we both knew it wasn't cancer. What could it be, and why wasn't he sharing?

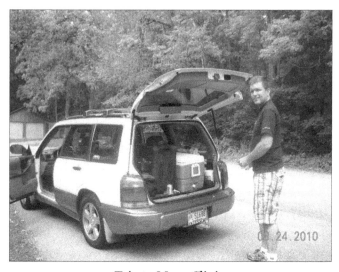

Trip to Mayo Clinic

Chapter 4

December 2010 capped off a year of major changes for us. I changed jobs, Steve stopped working, and to make sure we could survive the loss of Steve's income, we sold our three-bedroom spacious ranch home and downsized into a small mobile home with less than 1,000 square feet. Steve, Jacob, Emily, and I were suddenly living in close quarters in this small mobile home. Despite losing so much financially, we were happy. We knew it was the right time to recommit to each other, so Steve and I decided we wanted to renew our vows. When we married in 1988, we had eloped to Norfolk, Virginia, and got married by a justice of the peace. Since renewing our faith and marriage, we wanted to renew our vows in the church.

On a cold Saturday night, we said our vows in front of a small group of family and close friends in a candlelit ceremony at Rogers Creek Baptist Church, our small country church, with our Pastor Terry officiating. I helped Steve put on a white, button-down dress shirt and navy-blue dress pants. I wore a white button-down dress shirt, black pencil skirt, and my favorite black dress boots with a heel.

Our children, Jacob and Emily, stood next to us. Emily wore a red dress with glitter. Having hated wearing dresses after the age of five, this was a big deal for her. Jacob even dressed up in his white dress shirt and khaki carpenter jeans.

Steve refused to be seated during our vows and wanted to stand, even though his balance was so poor. He steadied himself by locking his arms and holding my hands as he stood for our vows. Terry read the vows to us: "I, Kim, take **you,** Steve, to be my husband, to have and behold from this day on, for better or for worse, for richer, for poorer, in sickness and in health, to love and to cherish, until death **do** us part."

"I do," I said with tears in my eyes. I meant it; I would cherish this man in his sickness—there would be no more health—and I would do it until death did us part and, ultimately, I did. These words were a driving force as his wife and caregiver.

As our renewed marriage began, Steve became less and less mobile, and our old way of life dwindled. At first, he tried to use a walker or hold onto my shoulders if we were walking short distances. We developed this makeshift walking system, where he would lock his arms and hold onto my shoulders from behind, and we would walk into church or very short distances. It enabled him to steady himself as he dragged his legs along, and we walked slowly. It kept the permanent use of the wheelchair at bay—temporarily. This system didn't last long.

One Sunday morning, as we were trying to walk into church, Steve fell backward, and all six feet, 200 pounds of him crashed onto the pavement in a thud. The other

Chapter 4

men at church ran to him and lifted him off the ground. That hurt his pride more than the bruises on his body.

Our makeshift way of walking was now a safety concern, and Steve decided it was time to move to the wheelchair. Steve was never able to return to work again after our return home from the Mayo Clinic. He had now been out of work less than a year.

Still believing he had Parkinson's disease, his first local neurologist prescribed an increasingly higher dose of Carbidopa Levodopa. However, the Carbidopa Levodopa seemed to barely touch the slight tremor he was having in his hand and offered no relief to any of the bladder or bowel problems. This seemed to be an aggressive case of Parkinson's disease. I knew several people with PD, and none of them seemed to transition to a wheelchair as quickly as Steve had. Though the initial diagnosis was Parkinson's disease, Steve continued to do his own research, and because of his lack of response to the traditional medications to control symptoms of Parkinson's disease, this led him to believe he might have a rare neurological disease called Multiple System Atrophy (MSA), which had similarities to Parkinson's. I had never even heard of this disease before.

A few years later, after multiple trips to the Mayo Clinic and visits with what seemed like hundreds of specialists, we started to get some answers to our questions about Steve's ever-increasing list of medical problems.

Though he suspected MSA, it took several lengthy trips to the Mayo Clinic before we got a definitive diagnosis. On the fourth trip, we were finally able to put a name to the mystery and learned Steve's original suspicion was correct.

Waiting for the neurologist that day, I sat desperately praying that he would tell us the name of this thing that was robbing Steve of his independence and livelihood. *Please, please, you have no idea what a name will mean,* I thought. *You have no idea how important this is to us just to know what we are facing.* For us, this was D Day, Diagnosis Day.

Dr. Dower, a tall, thin, dark-haired neurologist with glasses walked into his office and greeted us. His office was pleasant and included what he had described as a favorite painting of a farm, and, of course, the requisite picture of his family.

I sat on a small couch in the doctor's office while Steve stayed in his wheelchair, our knees touching, and our hands interlocked. Handholding was one of the few physical interactions we could continue to have with this terrible disease. We tried to hug but our connection was diminished with the wheelchair always getting between us like a toddler pining for our attention.

Dr. Dower had served as an officer in the Navy. Empathically, he had a great bedside manner and formed an instant connection with Steve. Though we were still relatively clueless, he knew what we would face for years to come; thus, his empathy for Steve.

Chapter 4

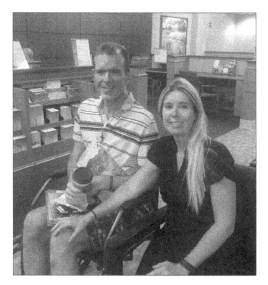

Steve and Kim Mayo Clinic

"How have things been going?" he asked Steve. "Can you tell me about any changes in your symptoms?"

By this point, Steve's voice had started to diminish. It required extra breath for him to talk, and his voice was just above a whisper. To compensate, he generally deferred to me to answer questions for him. I spoke up and started to answer Dr. Dower. "We have been noticing . . ."

"No, I want to hear from him," Dr. Dower said.

I was a little confused. Why would he want to make Steve go through such an effort when I knew his symptoms better than anyone? Of course, later I realized he was assessing a change in his symptoms and wanted to evaluate the loss of his voice.

As Steve had researched, Dr Dower confirmed that based on the extensive testing the Mayo Clinic had completed he likely had Multiple System Atrophy (MSA):

MSA is a rare neurodegenerative disorder that can cause a multitude of symptoms, including impairment to balance, difficulty with movement, poor coordination, bladder dysfunction, sleep disturbances, and poor blood pressure control. The disease was first known as Shy-Drager Syndrome.

In 1960, Dr. Milton Shy, assigned to the National Institute of Health, and Dr. Glen Drager, from Baylor College of Medicine in Houston, described in the Archives of Neurology two individual patients, who shared common clinical symptoms. Both patients were males who became sexually impotent and developed bladder problems at the ages of 39 and 49 respectively.

Their urinary problems became worse and within a very few months both patients complained of dizziness upon rising from either a sitting or lying positions which cause momentary "blackouts."

They later developed constipation, urinary and rectal incontinence, slowness of movement, unsteady gait, slurring of speech, mild tremors and other Parkinsonian symptoms. Upon examination, they had very low blood pressure when standing, and in addition to some Parkinsonian findings, they also had wasting of muscles in their hands and feet, dry skin due to loss of sweating and loss of pigment in the iris of the eyes.

Additional testing revealed abnormal function of the autonomic nervous system.

The second patient subsequently died and the postmortem examination provided evidence that he had a distinct and unique disease. Doctors Shy and Drager recognized that there was a link between low blood pressure during erect posture (orthostatic hypotension) and disturbances in the central autonomic system. To acknowledge their contribution, this disorder was named "Shy-Drager Syndrome" (SDS).

Today, Shy-Drager Syndrome (now known as Multiple System Atrophy) is a neurological disease resulting from degeneration of certain nerve cells in the brain and spinal cord. Body functions controlled by these areas of the brain and spinal cord function abnormally in patients with this disease. These include the autonomic nervous system or involuntary nervous system (which controls blood pressure, heart rate, and bladder function) and the motor system (control of balance and muscle movement). People in all parts of the world are affected, with onset usually between ages 45 and 60. As many as 50,000 Americans have this disease. The exact cause of the disease is not known. It is not inherited and it is not contagious.

Depending upon which part of the brain is affected first, the Multiple System Atrophy may appear in different ways. Sometimes it presents with low blood pressure on standing, urinary bladder problems, or difficulties with balance and movement that resemble Parkinson's disease.

Multiple System Atrophy is often difficult to treat because of the fluctuations in blood pressure. The general treatment course is aimed at controlling symptoms. Sleeping in a head-up position at night may reduce headaches and morning dizziness. An artificial feeding tube or breathing tube may be surgically inserted for management of swallowing and breathing difficulties.[1]

Dr. Dower was very careful not to provide a definitive diagnosis. He explained that only by examining the brain during autopsy could the disease be confirmed, so the best he could offer was a probable diagnosis. Through

---

[1] "The History of Multiple System Atrophy", Multiple System Atrophy Coalition, Accessed March 13, 2022. https://www.multiplesystematrophy.org/about-msa/history-multiple-system-atrophy-formerly-shy-drager-syndrome-sds/

our own research, we already knew there was no cure, and the disease would ultimately be terminal. There were only medications to manage symptoms. "Probable" was enough to give us a diagnosis.

It was very rare for someone his age to have the disease. It usually presents in people in their sixties; Steve started having initial symptoms in his thirties.

Hearing this diagnosis had the opposite effect that some might think. We didn't break down and cry; we didn't start making end-of-life plans; we didn't decide it was time to take that dream vacation we always wanted. We were just thankful to have a name and begin the journey. We didn't have time to think about the destination because we finally knew exactly what we were facing, or so we thought.

Ultimately, no matter how many doctors, books, or pamphlets prepare you, you never know exactly what you are facing. Steve was in his early forties at the time, and we were about to enter a dark world for which we felt ill-prepared. Looking back, I realize it was better we did not know the journey ahead.

Having a diagnosis emotionally helped both of us. Without a cure or treatment and only medications to help improve symptoms, however, the diagnosis was still devastating.

Most people typically live seven to ten years after initial symptoms, sometimes a little longer. Steve had already been having symptoms for about six years before he was diagnosed. He quickly realized he probably had three years at best, possibly five left to live.

He was better than me at recognizing this, as I absolutely blocked that news from my brain. I knew the information, yet I wasn't ready to accept what it meant. Steve looked at me and asked, "Can you handle this?" What he really meant was not could I handle the news but could I handle how hard this would become our marriage, our family, and me. "Of course, I can handle this," I naively said without reservation.

Life as we knew it was changing. Our roles in our marriage were changing. He could no longer take care of the kids and me, be the leader of our family, be the breadwinner, be my partner, or watch our children graduate, get married, and have kids.

I had two options: fight or flight. I immediately went into fight mode. It seemed to be a form of self-preservation, but I didn't allow myself any other option. It wasn't easy. I had never been a caregiver and had no idea what I was in for. In my opinion, I lacked the caregiver gene. The thought of being a caregiver was hard to embrace. I was impatient and more the "Hurry up and quit your whining about being sick" type of caregiver. It's not that I wasn't empathetic or caring. I was I just didn't want caregiving as a full-time job. Service was not my love language, as it felt completely foreign to my nature.

Once Steve broke a finger in a farming accident. To protect the finger, he had this giant cheese block-looking piece of foam on his entire hand. It got in the way so much he needed help taking a shower for a week. You would have thought I was being forced to march one hundred miles in the snow, wearing flip-flops while toting a family of polar bears on a sled. So inconvenienced did I feel having to help him with his shower. Such a minuscule amount of caregiving, and how well I had the nature then! So, you see, I was the last person to become Florence Nightingale!

During our marriage counseling, Steve and I had learned each other's love languages. I learned I identify best with physical touch and words of affirmation. Those are the ways I show love and best like to receive love, as they just come naturally to me. The love language I least identify with is quality time and acts of service. I like to have my alone time. After learning about my love language, being a resentful caregiver would soon make complete sense.

Caregiving was going to test my ability to learn how to sacrifice my independence and do everything for Steve, while at the same time losing the love language I so desperately needed: hearing how much he loved and cared about me and feeling him hug me. Still, I was going to do everything in my power to take care of him.

Now that we knew it was MSA, we absorbed every information we could get our hands-on. We read every bit of research we could find, joined every support group available on the internet, and talked to anyone else we found with the diagnosis, hungry for knowledge and hopeful for treatments. Unfortunately, we found more questions than answers. MSA affects every person a bit differently, and most of the doctors in our area had only heard of MSA in a textbook.

Each time we went to a medical appointment, had a procedure or test done, or met with a new doctor, it was like starting from scratch explaining MSA to the doctors. Also, many doctors immediately heard the MS in MSA and didn't realize it was an entirely different disease. To solve the problem, I prepared a one-page fact sheet that we took to each medical appointment. It described the disease, every medication he was taking, and any medications that were not recommended by his neurologist at the Mayo Clinic.

In the meantime, Rochester, Minnesota, became a place we visited regularly and continued to do so after the diagnosis. In the beginning, we made two trips a year to test medications, repeat tests, and follow his progress with specialists.

We learned to love Rochester. A beautiful and clean city, Rochester lies alongside the South Fork of the long Zumbro River and is ringed by gentle hills, farmland, and forests. We found the people warm and friendly for the most part. Usually, we stayed at the same Hampton Inn, which had a free shuttle service about fifteen minutes to the Mayo Clinic.

Having visited, unfortunately, often, I learned neighborhoods and recognized shuttle bus drivers and hotel staff. I even had a favorite restaurant, Culver's, known for their frozen custard. Each time we made a visit to Rochester, Culver's was one of our first stops for the delicious frozen treat.

Visits to the Mayo Clinic were the only form of "vacation" we had for the first five years that Steve was sick. While there, I embraced it for what it was. I took the art and history tour of the clinic while Steve was having a procedure done. To this day, I can tell you what types of art are displayed on each floor at the clinic.

While at the hotel, I would go for evening walks in the adjacent neighborhoods and imagine what it was like to be one of the happy families playing in their manicured

Chapter 4

yards along my walk. I would see dads playing ball with their kids and long for this sense of normalcy. During the weekends, I would drive Steve to go sightseeing around the area. He loved to be out on the road just riding around. Growing up in a family of long-distance truck drivers had given him the love of the open road.

I felt this sense of peace when we arrived at the rotunda of the Mayo Clinic, as if all our questions would have answers. I could feel a slight sense of happiness like we were somewhere where wheelchairs and sickness were not foreign but normal and acceptable. We rarely left with all the answers to our questions, but I knew we were at the one place in the world that likely had the most answers for his rare disease.

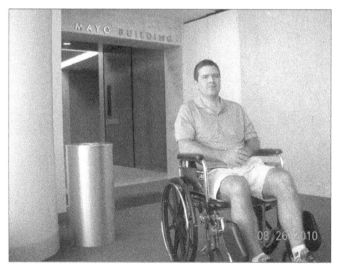

Steve at the Mayo Clinic

Chapter 5

Once Steve was diagnosed, our lives turned upside down. I had changed jobs, and we were unable to manage the farm anymore with Steve's failing health. Complicating things more was holding it together as parents of two young teenagers who were too consumed in their own lives to have any desire to be a part of the regular doctors' visits and trips to medical centers we had become immersed in.

At thirteen, Emily was in the throes of adolescence. Five-foot-three with long, chestnut, wavy hair, she was going through typical youth turbulence and started to distance herself from Steve and me. Initially, this seemed a normal teenage thing, as adolescence is the time of individuation and separation from parents. Emily had to figure out her own identity different from that of her parents.

With Emily, her distancing was extreme. Regularly angry and rarely smiling, regardless of what I said or did, she hid in her room, playing with her little chihuahua dogs Stan and Bella and listening to music.

She used to adore Steve and loved to help him on the farm and be a daddy's girl. One time, he gave her an abandoned calf to raise and feed. She named him Nacho and loved going with Steve daily to the farm to bottle-feed and hand-raise him.

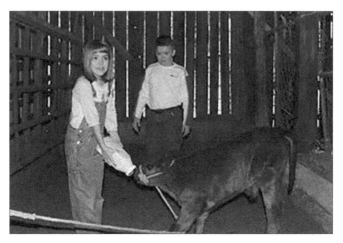

Emily, Jacob, and Nacho

Emily and I were closer. Unlike Jacob, she wanted to be around me more and disliked being alone. To accommodate her needs, I would take her with me when I could, for instance, to go shopping or, once when she was about ten, to get our nails done together. While she wasn't much on shopping, she would be happy as a lark if it included a visit to a pet store. One time, I took her for a surprise visit to a special pet store in Knoxville. They kept all the puppies in baby cribs specially designed for dogs. We simply walked around the store and held all the puppies. Emily was genuinely happy and talkative.

As a teenager, I encouraged her to be open with me about her feelings, thoughts, day, and so forth. I would reassure her that I would love her no matter what she did. I might not like the act, but I would still love her.

Nothing seemed to work. She just seemed to withdraw more and more. I soon realized this was likely the beginning stages of grief over having lost the father she knew.

Jacob was a different story. When he was born, Jacob was a happy baby who rarely cried and was generally in a good mood. He liked to play on his own a lot.

At the age of four, his preschool gave Jacob an evaluation for kindergarten. They suggested further evaluation because he was behind in speech. He generally did not communicate with more than his teacher and only when asked. He never initiated a conversation with anyone. When other adults at school would talk to him, he would blankly look without responding. From this evaluation, we learned Jacob had Asperger syndrome. Asperger syndrome is a condition on the autism spectrum, with most people considered being generally higher functioning, meaning they can talk, communicate, and participate in daily activities. Those with Asperger's may be socially awkward and have an all-absorbing interest in specific topics. For Jacob, this was video games and pro-wrestling.

Most people never knew about his diagnosis, nor did we share this information with many. It was complicated to explain. I had hoped they would think he was shy and quiet and treat him normally.

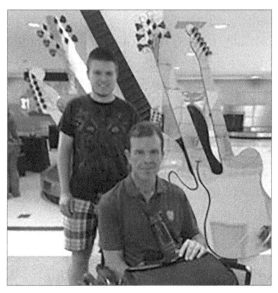

Jacob and Steve

Jacob would do anything I asked without complaint, which I thought was a byproduct of Asperger's. However, I think it is more his nature. Jacob is black and white about everything. If I provided specific, step-by-step instructions, he would provide help. As Steve became more dependent on help, Jacob became consumed with video games and liked to stay in his room. It was an escape for him, and I never questioned it.

Jacob and Emily rarely had friends over from school. Jacob had one friend from school named Zack and would occasionally ask to go to his house. Zack was a boy who lived up the road from us, tall and husky with dark hair. He had kind of a tough-kid appearance but was genuinely kind-hearted to Jacob. Zack had a younger brother who was developmentally delayed, and I think he empathized with Jacob's social isolation. Zack also had a tendency of getting into trouble at school if he hung around the wrong crowd. With Jacob, there was no chance of this happening, for he didn't follow the crowd and cause trouble. In their early teens, Jacob and Zack would play video games, watch movies, ride bikes, and go outside on adventures in the woods near our home.

Emily had few friends over as well. The only kids who ever visited were her cousins or an occasional friend from church. She kept her circle of friends very tight, and I am sure, in some ways, she was embarrassed to have friends over. The house was too small. Her tiny bedroom had enough room for her full-size bed, a dresser, and an old green armoire that held her TV and some of her games and mementos. With paper-thin walls and laminated fake wood-type doors that resembled more of Styrofoam bedrooms in an older model mobile home, they were not exactly the spacious rooms kids today might be used to. Other than their rooms, there was no escape from the wheelchair and their dad's disease. We had a small covered front porch if the weather was nice enough that the kids could sit on, but again, it was within inches of the front door, and their dad was almost permanently stationed nearby in the living room because it was one of the few places in the house his motorized wheelchair would fit, so there was no level of privacy.

Our lives were changing so drastically and felt like we were going in reverse, not progressing as most couples do. Gone were talk and dreams of a new car, vacations, a larger house, Steve gainfully employed, and the family financially comfortable.

During our entire marriage, we both worked full-time. The thought of either of us not working until retirement had never entered our minds. Now, Steve could no longer work. He could barely walk, no longer dress himself in the mornings, and had significant problems with urinary incontinence to where self-catheterization was necessary to go to the bathroom.

Daily, he suffered pounding headaches and debilitating, short-term memory loss intensified. The memory loss was a new challenge for us. Steve had the memory of an elephant. He never forgot a single detail about anything the whole time we were married. I rarely remembered the smallest detail, remembering only the important ones while tending to look at the big picture. This disparity caused a few arguments over the years.

One time, one of Steve's wrenches came up missing from the garage, and I had recently used it to fix something in the house. The garage was in such disarray I had no idea where the darn thing was. I probably laid it down near where it was supposed to go, but I couldn't remember exactly where I put it. Needless to say, I immediately decided to purchase a small set of tools for myself to keep in the house. Now I wasn't the only one who couldn't remember all the details. Finally, we were equals!

I had been at my new job for less than a year. With Steve not working, our finances would soon be severely strained, and we were unprepared. Who prepares for their husband getting a dreaded, can't-be-cured, fatal disease!

Though we both had good jobs, we, like so many, had lived outside our means and survived paycheck to paycheck. We had always talked about saving, but for some reason, we have never made it a reality, just a dream. Saving money was now the furthest of our problems.

The first month of Steve's lost income, we struggled to make our mortgage payment, put gas in the car, pay the utility bills, and buy groceries. What would the coming months be like? I couldn't begin to even think about our future.

A few years back, we had bought a piece of property with a small mobile home on it. Our hope was that someday, we would build a house on this land. Now our only hope was that we could continue to make payments on both the land with the mobile home and the mortgage payment on our current home until it sold.

I was mad at both of us. We were about to face a crisis we should have planned for and didn't. How am I going to tell my boss I can't make it to work because I can't afford to fix my car, even though I am earning a decent middle-class wage? Humbled by my situation, I realized you never know what lies behind a façade of happiness.

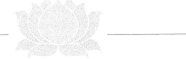

Chapter 6

Not long after we lost Steve's income, we had to sell our home, downsize, and move into the mobile home on the property we owned. We couldn't afford to make both the mortgage payment on our home and pay on the property we owned any longer.

We had been living in a 1,500 square-foot three-bedroom, one-bath home with a huge kitchen and pantry, and a large, unfinished addition to the house that was added before we bought it. We never finished it, but it made for great storage space.

Now we had to move into a three-bedroom mobile home barely 1,000 square feet. We had made some improvements to it over the past couple of years, so I tried to be optimistic. It was small, so that meant less house to clean. The kitchen and living room were basically one room—I had always told Steve I wanted an open concept kitchen and living space. Be careful what you wish for! In truth, the kitchen was so tiny there was barely room to store any dishes, let alone food.

My life seemed to be going backward. Before Steve got sick, I thought we were on a life trajectory to continue working hard, save for the future, and maybe build a house of our own someday. We had always talked about building a house. For years, Steve had saved magazine articles about construction trends, design styles, and innovative features. Now instead, we were boxing up those magazine articles for storage and downsizing into a mobile home.

This bothered me because my mom grew up very poor. I didn't quite appreciate her definition of very poor when I was young. I think all parents tell their kids how poor they were when they were younger; however, as I got older, I realized she was not exaggerating. Her father had built their house on a small piece of land mostly out of cinder blocks and basic framed walls. There were few walls with insulation, and most walls didn't have drywall or paneling. In northern Ohio, I can only imagine how cold it was in the winter. Probably of most significance, her family had an outhouse. She was the oldest of six kids and never had a toilet, shower, or hot water.

We, of course, had all those things growing up and didn't lack for anything essential because my dad worked for the electric company. For the most part, my mom stayed home with my two younger sisters and me, as women at that time were expected to do. Occasionally, she worked in an office or department store when we needed extra money to pay bills.

Still, I knew my family had money worries. We didn't have savings, usually owned an older used car, and rarely, if ever, went out to eat. We never took a vacation except to visit family.

My mom would pack a picnic lunch of very thin-sliced chipped-chopped ham sandwiches on hoagie buns that

Chapter 6

she got from the deli and some store-brand potato chips. We would each get to pick out our favorite flavor of off-brand soda. Mine was always orange.

Usually, we would visit my great-grandfather, who lived alone about two hours south in an old Victorian house in Marion, Ohio. If we weren't visiting him, we would sometimes go to Lake Erie near Cleveland and sit on the rocky sand beach and play. The water was cold coming off Lake Erie, but it was the closest I had ever been to a real beach. These were my favorite times of childhood. It's hard to miss what you have never had!

The day I turned sixteen, the legal working age in Ohio at the time, I got my first job at Vaccaro's Italian Restaurant in the kitchen. I was responsible for keeping the massive salad bar refilled and cleaned. I wanted to have money to buy a car, hang out with friends, and have my independence.

After I started working, I paid all my expenses. I bought an old Ford Mustang, gas, money for food, and essentials. To help my parents out, I even bought a screen door for our house when ours broke. While in college, I worked part-time for extra money in the cash office at a regional grocery called Apple's Grocery Store near my house.

Chapter 7

The financial strain of Steve no longer working and medical co-payments increasing continued to bother me. Now I felt our family was going back to those pinching pennies days of my early life. As a mother, it was upsetting. I had tried to make sure Jacob and Emily never felt our problems. We weren't rich, but they would never lack. However, with Steve disabled and no longer working, I wasn't sure I could guarantee that level of comfortable living.

If we were middle class, our situation didn't reflect it. The world mirrored this realization as I began to understand what it must look like to outsiders that we were moving from our current home to the *mobile home*. Downsizing was an understatement.

When we moved, I hired a local moving company to move our furniture. Steve could not help at all from his wheelchair.

I had planned for the move and set aside the $400 it was going to cost to move all the furniture and appliances. When the moving company was finished, the owner asked to talk to me outside. Sheepishly, he explained that they would be willing to provide a discount if I needed one because they liked to help members of the community in need.

I was caught off guard. How did he know how bad of a financial strain we were under right then? I thanked him for the offer but told him I had the money to pay for the move. I was the only one in the neighborhood who didn't see how bad it was.

Well, not quite. I felt it every time we went to the grocery store. We used to buy what we wanted. While not extravagant, neither did we worry if we spent too much. Now, with a limited budget, I suddenly yearned for that name-brand cereal that I wouldn't have thought twice about buying before.

When we went to the grocery store, I tried to be creative. Jacob and Emily's request for potato chips was met with off-brand saltine crackers. Soda turned into unsweetened powdered drink packets. Hamburgers for dinner? No, thank you, we love rice and beans!

The grocery store trips slapped the kids with the reality that our lives had changed drastically. They knew Dad was sick, but not in a "this terminal illness is going to drain us financially" kind of way.

Poor Emily really felt the brunt of it. She was taking an agricultural class in high school, where students had an opportunity to purchase a piglet through the class and raise it at home. Emily has a tremendous love for animals. If money, time, and my permission were no object, she would have her own Noah's Ark on our property.

I barely remember the conversation where she asked if she could get a pig. I think I said, "We can't do that." In my mind, that meant I don't have the ability to build a pen

Chapter 7

for it; Dad can't help, as he is in a wheelchair, and in all likelihood, it would be one more pet for me to have to feed, worry about, and take care of. Maybe in my usual multitasking and haste to accomplish too many things at once, I answered her with an "Emily, we can't afford a pig."

I went on and forgot about the conversation, that is until the school called me at work one day. After her mother crushed her hopes of becoming a pig farmer, Emily went to school and told her teacher her family could not afford a pig. This is a fairly small farming community, and we knew many of the teachers at the high school. They knew Steve. They knew that Steve and his whole family had always farmed.

With him being a disabled veteran in a wheelchair, the teachers wanted to help. Since Emily told them her family couldn't afford to purchase a piglet, the teachers generously offered to pool their own money and buy the pig for us. As a mom, this touched my heart. As a caregiver, working mom, and the person responsible for everything in our family, this terrified me. Ultimately, we thanked the school for their generosity but decided pig farming was probably a little more than we could handle now.

Emily was crushed, and I felt so guilty for having to say no to the pig. If I could have been honest about everything we were facing, maybe she would have understood, but how was I going to tell a thirteen-year-old, "Hey, there's a good chance your dad is not going to see you graduate from high school because he is going to get worse, not better." Pig farming was the least of our problems. The thought that Steve might not see Emily graduate was more prophetic than I could have realized.

Chapter 8

Living with Steve day in and day out, I saw a little bit of change happening every day and didn't notice the dramatic change. I was living in la-la land. Surely, I knew he would only get worse, but I didn't see what I didn't want to see.

At home, some friends gave us a motorized scooter to use. It was a big help for Steve to use around the house, as our home was not very wheelchair-accessible. Steve could now only make it into the living room, bedroom, and hallway but not into the kids' rooms.

Emily's bedroom was down a narrow hallway, lined with wire utility shelves holding all of my pots, pans, and pantry items. Our kitchen was too tiny to hold much beyond our dishes and cups. Because of the narrow hallway, Steve could never get to her room. As a moody teenager, this was a plus for her.

Jacob's room was down the hallway from our room. Steve could ride his scooter down to it, but the doorway wasn't wide enough for him to get through. Besides, once he made it to Jacob's bedroom, there was no way to turn the scooter around, and he would have to back down the hallway.

The tiny bathroom we used became a bad version of Mr. Twister as we tried to negotiate how to get him in. As a caregiver, I learned how to bend at my knees to utilize the strength in my legs and pull him up using my arm strength, bracing his elbow and bicep in my hands to avoid straining my back. This allowed us to pivot him from the wheelchair into the bathroom.

We had a difficult time even shutting the bathroom door because I would have had to move his wheelchair out of the way to shut the door, and the bathroom was so small, the door opened into the hallway. This meant I would have to let go of Steve and, of course, I couldn't. So, modesty was completely out the door, literally at this point.

Early on, before we moved into this mobile home, Steve had metal handicap grab bars installed everywhere there was room. At the time, I thought it was completely unnecessary; now I was thankful for his foresight. He would hold onto the grab bar to steady himself while I prepared the intermittent urinary catheter on the small, narrow shelf above the toilet.

The first time I had to catheterize him with an intermittent catheter was traumatizing. The doctor taught him how to do it at first, but within six months, Steve could no longer catheterize himself, and I took over. It requires tremendous coordination and steadiness to clean everything, open up the packaging to the catheter, and perform the process. Steve was anything but coordinated and steady at this point.

Since Steve couldn't do much for himself and plenty of time on his hands at home to do research, he read every document the Veterans Administration made available regarding potential benefits for disabled veterans. He hoped this would help make up for his loss of income from not being able to work and supplement his health insurance.

Steve's neurologist told us that MSA is triggered in different ways. The first is genetic. This was ruled out, as Steve had no family history of it and had extensive genetic testing at the Mayo Clinic. Additionally, MSA might be brought on by traumatic brain injuries. This was ruled out because he had not had any.

Chemical exposure was the likely cause. While serving on board the ship in the electrical rewind shop while in the Navy many years earlier, Steve had extensive exposure to trichloroethylene, a chemical compound commonly used as an industrial solvent. In his research, Steve had found a similar case of MSA in a sailor in the Royal Navy who had heavy exposure to trichloroethylene.

We made regular, quarterly visits to the VA hospital, nearly three hours away from our house. There, Steve met with a neurologist in addition to the neurologist at the Mayo Clinic. This was important because the VA neurologist could authorize the medication Steve needed and provide the catheters and supplies at no charge to us. As the cost of medical bills and supplies increased, this was a huge blessing.

After almost two years in the scooter, Steve's neurologist at the Veteran's Administration (VA) referred him to the physical therapy department to be evaluated for a motorized wheelchair provided by the VA. To me, this wasn't even a question because Steve could not walk, but anything that happened through the VA required lots of layers of approvals and evaluations, and—most of the time—unfortunately, time was the one thing we lacked as Steve's disease progressed rapidly.

What an exciting day when the technician came to deliver and set up Steve's new wheelchair. It had a candy-apple red base with black trim and tilted and raised. Most importantly, it had an easy toggle switch that Steve could use to drive himself. However, the very touchy toggle switch combined with his lack of coordination from MSA equaled scarred walls and doors. Our poor house looked like someone inebriated had driven a dump truck up and down the hallways. I tried touch-up paint several times, but after a while, it became futile, and I gave up.

Finances were still tight. We needed a wheelchair van to allow Steve to use his wheelchair when we went somewhere, but we couldn't afford a new vehicle. Instead, we traveled everywhere in our white Subaru Forester with more than 300,000 miles on it and brought the transport wheelchair. Out of seven trips to the Mayo Clinic, five of them were made in the Forester. We improvised accessibility wherever possible.

How hard it was to transport someone in a wheelchair and get them in and out of a vehicle was something I never realized until now. I had no choice but to learn to carefully pull him out of the chair to a standing position, steady myself and him, and then pivot him to the car.

I had to get him in the correct placement in the seat; otherwise, I would have to push or pull him into place. Once his bottom was in the seat, I pulled his legs, one by

Chapter 8

one, up and into the car, reached over and buckled his seatbelt, and sealed the transaction with a kiss.

We traveled with a lightweight transfer chair so that I could put it in the back and get it out by myself. In this way, I could transport Steve without having to lug his motorized wheelchair along.

Any type of travel became very difficult, as it meant we had to double or triple the amount of time for anything we did. If I was going to the store alone, getting dressed and walking out the door took fifteen minutes. Taking Steve out the door was another matter.

To start, it meant getting him dressed in his outfit of choice. Dressing a six-foot-tall, 200-pound, disabled man was like dressing an adult toddler, and it took so much time because Steve had a sense of style and refused to wear sweatpants or lounge pants anywhere in public. This had been a long-standing, agreed-upon rule in our marriage. As the Southern saying goes, "We would dress like we were somebody" when we were in public. While he didn't have to be dressed up, he did prefer to wear his Levi jeans whenever possible.

Dressing him in his Levi jeans further exhausted me and increased my frustration at having to take him. So much for looking for accessibility. This task should be added to pre-marital counseling to determine an engaged couple's true level of commitment to each other. That would quickly weed out loads of people not ready for marriage "in *sickness* and in health."

Next came the supplies needed on our short trip to the store. I had to first estimate the time we would be gone so I could pack the appropriate amount of medicines needed.

Steve took more than fifty pills each day and would have to take his carbidopa levodopa every 2.5 hours.

We packed an adult version of what Steve referred to as his diaper bag. It contained special, self-containing, intermittent catheter supplies, water bottles, wipes, and extra medicine just in case.

Now we began the process of actually getting Steve into the car. If he rode his motorized scooter to the car, I would have to ride his scooter back into the house after I got him safely in the car.

After this whole endeavor, I was about to collapse. On top of that, I had to do the driving and start this whole circus over again once we got to the store or wherever we were going.

I did it with a smile. I did so even when Steve, having gone stir crazy in our tiny house during the day, insisted on going out after I arrived home totally exhausted from a day's work and commuting an hour each way back and forth. It didn't matter if it was the grocery store, out to eat, or just looking around Walmart. He wanted out of this small mobile home that had become his prison, minus bars, from the outside world.

Though I wanted nothing more than to park the car and chill on the couch staring at the TV, I agreed as I sympathized with his feeling trapped. After being able to drive anywhere, my heart went out to what it must have been like for him to now be dependent on me to make this happen.

Chapter 8

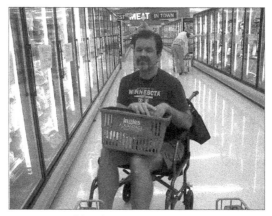

Steve in one of his favorite places the grocery store

Still, the situation brought up so many emotions for me. I was exhausted to the bone and didn't feel like Steve understood that, causing some tension between us. At the same time, I felt guilty for putting my own need for rest first. I knew I could rest someday, but he could never drive where he wanted to.

Seventeen at the time, Jacob willingly helped me do everything and didn't turn me down if I asked him to take his dad or help me, but I felt tremendous guilt for the burden that placed on Jacob. I didn't think it was fair to Jacob to take over as a caregiver for his dad for me at times.

Emily was almost sixteen and seemed to despise caring for her dad in any fashion. She helped, but I knew she didn't want to. I recognized this now as grief. For Emily, it was her way of coping with losing the dad she knew. She started disconnecting from him years before he died she later told me because, in her mind, the dad she knew was already dead.

With my own exhaustion and how caring for Steve impacted the children, I desperately wished for someone, anyone, to rescue me from this growing caregiving hell. Ultimately, I coped by compartmentalizing my feelings of anger, frustration, grief, and exhaustion. If I was having a bad day and about to collapse from exhaustion, I told my brain not to go there. I didn't have the time or energy to be exhausted.

On the days I drove to work crying, I would create things to say to my coworkers. I knew they were going to ask how Steve was doing or how I was doing. I couldn't bear to open up the emotional river that would happen if I was honest. Quickly I learned that not everyone wants to know how you are doing. They just want to be able to say they've asked. I know others wanted to help, but they just didn't know how. I would come to realize that not everyone is comfortable enough to have the hard conversations about the reality of disease and the discussion about how difficult it is.

I also became adept at turning the conversation to something else. I would say something like, "I'm doing okay. Steve is doing okay. We are tremendously blessed. Why don't you tell me about what is going on in your family?" Or I would say in a joking manner, "I'm exhausted right now but can't wait for the weekend to catch up." In truth, I hated the weekend. It meant no escape from the caregiving—no drive to work to cry my heart out.

Chapter 9

We had been living in our tiny mobile home for a couple of years. Steve was now too debilitated to stand unassisted at all and was confined to a wheelchair. Despite this, he tried to maintain as much independence as possible.

Each day, he tried to transfer himself from his wheelchair to the toilet seat. There was little in the way of handicap bars in our tiny house. We had tried to add them, but wall space is limited in a mobile home, and it's difficult to find a sturdy place to adhere a metal handicap grab bar. The one we did have in the bathroom was on the other side of the toilet, so Steve leveraged himself on the arm of his motorized wheelchair. Many times, that was to my detriment; one particular night, I remember.

Balance and sleep were a few of the areas that MSA robbed from Steve. One night, when he was too restless to fall sleep, he decided to get up on his own and go to the living room to read or watch TV.

To help get Steve in and out of bed, we had placed a large metal, trapeze-style device next to the bed and handrails on the bed. I always parked Steve's motorized wheelchair right next to the bed to make it easier to get him in and out of bed.

That night, I was in a comatose state and never heard Steve manage to pull himself out of bed, slide into the wheelchair, and somehow sneak out of the bedroom. Despite his balance, he still had some strength in his arms and used it to pull himself up whenever he could. He didn't make it far, thanks to his motorized wheelchair I affectionately called "Christine."

Christine hated me for some reason. She regularly showed off by pinning me in precarious situations. One example was the time I tried to help guide Steve out the back door and down the slight wheelchair ramp onto the small concrete walkway at the back door. I was standing near him in my shorts and flip-flops, not paying attention, when Christine drove straight toward my big toe and nearly tore off my toenail. "That hurt," I screamed!

Steve had a grin on his face. If I didn't know better, I would have thought he was intentionally laughing. Although, it was a weird side effect of MSA and out of his control. Sometimes he would laugh or cry at inappropriate times.

One evening, I was standing near the headboard of our bed, preparing to transfer Steve out of his wheelchair and into bed. Christine had other plans. As he got close to the bed, he bumped the toggle-type switch he used to operate the motorized wheelchair. For reasons I still do not understand, he seemed to be pushing the toggle switch right toward me. In a slow-motion kind of wheelchair collision, Christine kept slowly pushing me into the wall near our headboard.

Chapter 9

At first, I thought Steve was joking with me. Then I realized he couldn't get the toggle switch to go backward, and the wheelchair kept slowly pinning me harder against the wall. There was nowhere for me to move out of the way for my safety. My laughter soon turned into a panic at the thought of the rescue squad having to come to our house to dislodge a 250-pound wheelchair off me.

"Jacob!" I screamed. Now seventeen, Jacob lacked a panic button. He made his way at a normal pace to our room but didn't exactly sprint like I thought he would. At six feet, 200 pounds, Jacob, thankfully, had the strength of an ox and pulled the deadly wheelchair backward so I could escape. Somehow, this wheelchair seemed like a protective dog over her master, and she didn't want me around.

Another night, Christine showed off as usual. I think her mission was to make sure I didn't sleep. In Steve's not-so-subtle attempt to sneak out, Christine caught the door frame on their way out of the bedroom. A motorized wheelchair could be a powerful transportation device. Steve's wheelchair weighed around 250 pounds. Add power to that, an uncoordinated driver, dark conditions, and you have a recipe for destruction.

I woke up to the sound of our bedroom doorframe being ripped off the wall and dragged down the hallway. The sound of a door frames being torn off the hinges was a little unsettling at four in the morning.

Even that wasn't good enough for Christine. Apparently, we weren't stopping at one doorframe. Before I could gather my thoughts and get out of bed, Steve was headed to the bathroom. By the time I got the wheelchair stopped,

Christine had pushed right on through to the bathroom door and ripped it completely off its hinges. After one big sigh, I picked it up and sat in the hallway next to the bathroom in a trance. My day was starting off great.

In addition to waking me up from my precious few hours of sleep, I was stuck with figuring out how to do carpentry and repair these doors at 4 a.m.

I wanted to get mad. I really did, but how do you get mad at a guy who tried to be independent and let me sleep but quite unintentionally created huge problems for me? You can't. In fact, one had to admire my wheelchair-bound husband's Superman powers. He may not have been able to leap tall buildings, but he could tear two doors off their hinges in one short wheelchair roll through the hallway in the middle of the night!

Clearly, my day was off to a rough start, another night with only four hours of sleep. How did I survive it? I pushed forward by using my caregiving compartmentalizing skills; I shut out thoughts of frustration as soon as they crept into my mind and pressed on with my day.

I have no carpentry skills, so the best solution I could come up with was to sit the door in front of the bathroom when Steve had to use it. However, this temporary solution only worked if I picked up the door and sat it in front of the bathroom so Steve could have some privacy while he was in there. Now on top of having to physically take Steve to the bathroom, I was also the bathroom attendant.

Thankfully, we had a second bathroom that I could use. This bathroom was in a hallway that was not wheelchair-accessible, and Steve could not get into it. For our bedroom, we would just do without a door.

Chapter 9

The next morning, I called his brother Mike for some emergency bathroom door repair. Mike was one of those people I could always count on to help, and he had the door fixed in a jiffy.

Steve and Mike had always been close. Once Steve became sick, Mike became even closer to us. Anything that needed to be repaired or fixed, Mike would take care of. He was one of the only people brave enough to take Steve out on his own when I was working. He would load up Steve in the car and take him out to eat for a hamburger and French fries at Hardee's or just for a drive around. Steve liked to order food, but he could barely eat it since he was increasingly having more trouble swallowing food and clearing his throat, but at least he could get out and about.

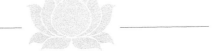

Chapter 10

For months, Steve had been asking me to look for a seat for an old truck we were having redone to replace our Subaru Forester. It was a 1977 orange Ford F100, in great shape with low miles. We called it the "pumpkin truck."

Having inherited the pumpkin colored truck from his dad years ago, Steve had dreamed of repainting and making it show-worthy. He collected catalogs on car parts, researched techniques and colors on the Internet, and watched shows to determine the latest trends.

Shortly after we made our first trip to the Mayo Clinic, Steve found someone who could restore this beautiful truck; that was in late 2010. On a Sunday afternoon, Steve drove the truck to the shop. It was a significant moment because it was probably one of the last times he drove and, most importantly, it was the last time he ever drove the truck. In six months, he would be in a wheelchair and unable to walk anymore.

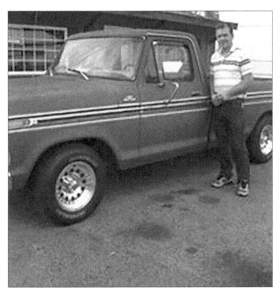

Steve and his dads 1977 Ford F100

Back to looking for a seat, I drove near the used auto parts warehouse but then decided to skip it. I didn't want to look for these seats and was out of my territory. I didn't know the first thing about auto parts, new or used, but this was one of many duties added into my caregiver role since Steve was now a couple of years into his diagnosis of MSA and experiencing increased muscle loss. He went through periods of no change that we referred to as a plateau. Then suddenly, he would experience a drop-down in his abilities. Now he was unable to do much of anything on his own, let alone drive.

Since the junkyard was an hour from our home, it was easier for me to stop on my way home than it was to go home, get Steve, and make a separate trip. Besides, I could never push Steve's wheelchair through the grass to let him decide. *I'd better suck it up,* I thought, *and go do this.*

I turned around and stopped at the junkyard on my way home from work. When else would I have a minute of free time? Did my coworkers have any clue what endeavors I went through? It's not like I walked out of my corporate job and said, "Have a good night. I'm heading to the junkyard on my way home because it's not wheelchair-accessible, and you know my husband is unable to walk anymore."

Who does that?

I pulled up to the junkyard, trembling. *How am I going to pretend I have even a clue about what I am doing? I am so out of my element here in a suit jacket and skirt; not exactly appropriate junkyard attire.*

Before me laid lots of junk cars, remnants of crashed vehicles, and dirt and weeds as far as I could see. I'd better dress down a notch before they laugh at me. Thankfully, it was a warm day, so I ditched the suit jacket and threw on a pair of flip-flops. Great, the only flip-flops with me were my glitter flip-flops, the kind an eight-year-old wears to the beach.

Several people greeted me behind a desk. They seemed friendly and not too judgmental of me. Maybe this wouldn't be so bad. I had my notes, and I could tell them what I needed. Hopefully, they would have mercy on me and get me what I needed without me having to trek through the weeds and grease of this junkyard.

Not so fast.

"I'm here to pick out a set of seats," I said to the scruffy-looking guy behind the counter, with long, wild black hair and tattoos down his arms.

"Okay," he said," Go out on the lot to look at the seats." He told me what vehicles to look for.

If you were a guy, this whole scenario would be like a kid in a candy store—perusing through wrecked cars in various states of disrepair, looking at all the available parts.

I was a fish out of water here. I looked down at my glittery flip-flops. *Should I tell him that I didn't care what the seats look like? Just get me one so I can leave without too much trauma.* My blank stare, along with my business suit, must have convinced him I was a damsel in distress, and he sent me out with a chatty young guy to lead the way.

He walked me through the garage bays and out to the junkyard. It was at least 150 degrees in the garage bays and filled with more dirt and grease than I had seen in a lifetime.

We made our way out to the junkyard. It was a plethora of organized used auto parts. How I regretted having worn a skirt and sparkly flip-flops. They were going to be anything but sparkly after I trekked around this junkyard.

Finally, after about an hour of viewing seats in various states of disrepair, and with some negotiating, I located and purchased the seats Steve needed. How awesome. I had survived my first trip to the junkyard and faced one of my fears. One item I had never had on my bucket list of life could officially be checked off—perusing a filthy junkyard in a business suit and glittery flip-flops.

Chapter 10

I returned home to my second job of the day as caregiver, only to learn I was to become an ad-hoc electrician that night. A lightning storm damaged the signal amplifier for the TV antennae. This wonderful little invention was in the attic. Steve told me we would need to replace the amplifier, and since the attic, with its drop-down ladder, was not wheelchair-accessible, it was on me.

At first, I whined in the usual fashion. "I am not an electrician. I don't know a thing about doing any of this." Both a blessing and a curse, my husband was extremely intelligent. He somehow believed his ability to read technical manuals and understand complex technology would be easy to explain to me. Maybe it would be if we were dealing with a normal situation, but we were dealing with a terminal illness that had robbed his ability to speak while keeping his intellect perfectly intact.

One of the many functions that MSA had robbed from Steve's body was speaking. Over the last few years, Steve's speech had become so soft it was just a step above a whisper. Now his breathing had become more difficult too. Steve found it hard to push air through his vocal cords to talk and had to take a deep breath to push the sound out. Conditions affecting breathing are common with MSA. They may arise from atrophy, over-activation of breathing or vocal cord muscles, or a combination of the two, as well as from degeneration in areas of the brain that control respiration.

Because the breathing difficulties interfered with his ability to speak, we developed a couple of methods of communication. When Steve needed something, he had a little brass bell he would ring. Like Pavlov's dogs, after a while, that bell would send a shiver down my spine because it meant the end of any chance to rest.

We also needed a way for him to tell me things without typing them out on his computer. I bought a piece of foam board about 11 18 at the dollar store and added a makeshift keyboard of stick-on black block letters. Steve could run his fingers over the letters and briefly pause long enough for me to write down the letters on a notepad and form sentences. As helpful as this was to communicate, it was painfully slow, and sometimes Steve would get confused while trying to say a long sentence and add in words or letters that didn't make sense.

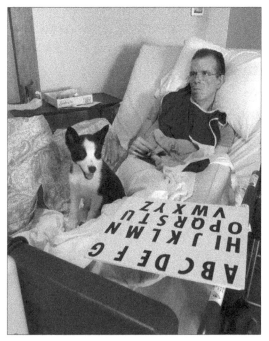

Steve and our makeshift communication board

Chapter 10

I hated this problem of trying to communicate. Hated it! I wanted desperately to carry on a conversation with my husband, but the one man in the world I wanted most to talk to couldn't converse with me. Most of our conversations were one-sided. I talked, and he added in a few words. To complicate things, the more I talked, the more he wanted to contribute, and it was so hard for him to do so.

Usually, I tried to keep conversations to a minimum to reduce the strain on him to talk and the effort it would require for me to listen.

Steve and I have been avid fans of the Dr. Phil Show and watch it religiously for advice and discussion topics. I've heard endless complaints on the Dr. Phil Show of how people don't listen to each other, but my dilemma gave a whole new meaning to "it takes effort for me to listen."

Of course, I had no choice but to put in that effort as I had become Steve's interpreter. His mom and brother Mike, who always helped when Steve needed anything, had begun to rely on me to translate because you had to press your ear very close to his mouth to hear what he was saying. It could take thirty minutes to get even a short sentence out. By then, you would be worn out from the strain. Most conversations with family and friends ended up with "Kim, can you tell me what he is saying?"

Exhausted and irritable, here I was leaning over his wheelchair with my ear pressed to almost his mouth as he instructed me laboriously in whispers in his slow, drawn-out manner, with my legs about to collapse.

Back to our antennae issue, listening to Steve was the only way I was going to figure out how to replace the amplifier in the attic, as this was something I was completely unequipped to do. When he said a few words, I had to repeat back what I heard to make sure I got it. I had to; there were no alternatives. If I didn't attempt this, it meant no TV stations at all on our bedroom TV. Once again, I sucked it up and gave it a try.

I made my way up to the unfinished attic and negotiated the roofing frame and the insulation. There was no flooring, just the framing. It was only about 4,000 degrees in the attic. In addition, for some reason, wasps seem to love the hot air; apparently, the hotter, the better.

I had no idea what the amplifier was, so I made an educated guess based on the wires coming in.

I thought I had located it, but I didn't see how I could replace it. It was solidly bolted in. Just to be sure, I whipped out my phone and took a picture to show Steve. I described it at length: the wires coming in, the wires going out, what it looked like, and how I checked everything.

He had no idea what I was describing. Suddenly, he burst out laughing. I was trying to disconnect and repair the speaker to the house alarm system, not the amplifier to the antennae.

I headed back up to the attic now that I knew which thing with wires was the amplifier. I called Jacob and Emily up to the attic to watch Mom practice home repair and replace the amplifier. I felt like I had a duty to teach them since Dad was unable. They could care less, but they needed to learn home improvement.

After I fended off the wasps that were now attracted to me because I was dripping with sweat, I maneuvered my

Chapter 10

way back over the rafters, gently avoided the insulation, and succeeded in not falling through the ceiling.

I was psyched when I completed the task of replacing the TV antennae amplifier in the attic. Maybe we should rewire the house! Next item off the bucket list of things I never wanted to accomplish.

Chapter 11

It had been four years since my life as a caregiver began and irrevocably changed all our lives.

"How do you do it?" my sister Michelle asked me. "How do you handle commuting to work one hour each way, working full time, being a full-time caretaker, kids, being active in church, the dogs, and fitting life in the middle somewhere?"

"I don't know. Some days I think I'm one spilled smoothie away from a nervous breakdown."

This became my battle cry after the blueberry smoothie incident.

I was running late for a credit union conference I was attending for work in Nashville, a two-and-a-half-hour drive from my house. I should have declined this meeting, but I tried to keep one foot in the door with work while trying to balance life at home. Most days, I was holding on like someone hanging off the edge of a cliff.

Normally, I would spend the night if I was attending a full-day meeting in Nashville. Instead, I decided to attempt the trip in one day, adding to the anxiety of the morning. After putting on my black business pencil skirt suit with a matching blazer, a white button-up blouse, and my favorite, black, zip-up, dressy-heeled boots, I did a quick makeup routine of foundation, mascara, and a little blush. I love jewelry, so I added my silver hoop earrings and favorite silver cross necklace. Thankfully, I was able to quickly pull back my hair into a ponytail.

    I made my way to our tiny kitchen to make Steve a smoothie. We daily made smoothies because Steve had difficulty swallowing, so soft foods worked best. I pulled the blueberries and milk out of the refrigerator and mixed them on the counter with the small blender. The blender was one of the few appliances we had room for on the tiny counter space, at least a quarter of it covered with medicine bottles, syringes, a heavy -duty pill crusher, containers for mixing medicine, and various medical supplies.

    With MSA, many of the muscles begin to atrophy, and swallowing becomes arduous. Most foods would cause Steve to choke, and that, in turn, could cause aspiration pneumonia. During one of his recent hospital stays, Steve's doctor advised that he should have a feeding tube placed in his stomach. He had been unable to consume solid foods for almost a week, and his doctor told us it was only a matter of time before it was absolutely required.

    His doctors and I naively thought this would remedy Steve's swallowing problems because he would receive all his nutrition through his feeding tube and have no need to eat actual food. But he still wanted to eat. Despite downing cartons of liquid nutrition each day via his feeding tube, he still craved eating and all things food.

    He watched cooking shows and the Food Network incessantly. At one point, I was convinced he was in love with Food Network star Ree Drummond because he watched her shows so much. He loved collecting recipes for meals he couldn't cook or eat, and he loved to look at cookbooks and turn down pages to mark recipes.

His nutrition doctor at the Mayo Clinic explained to us that this phenomenon was studied during World War II in something called the Minnesota Starvation Experiment[2]. Conscientious objectors were deprived of food to help researchers determine how to treat victims of mass starvation. The researchers learned that the men craved food so much when they couldn't eat that they would stand outside of restaurants to watch people eating inside. This made so much sense now. Steve loved to have food in front of him, even if he couldn't eat it.

Steve's balance continued to get much worse, and as I finished getting ready to leave after giving him his smoothie, Steve was standing, bracing himself between the wheelchair and counter. He held onto the counter to keep strength in his muscles. However, his muscles were never as strong as he thought they were, and he and the smoothie soon fell. The giant glass of blueberry smoothie flew out of his hand, hit the floor, splashed up on the ceiling, the walls, and my freshly pressed black dress suit and back all over the floor where Steve was lying. He was laughing. As mentioned, laughing, or crying at inappropriate times was a side effect of MSA.

I wanted to scream at him for falling! How thoughtless of him to fall and spill a smoothie while I was trying to get out the door for work. I was so angry! Realizing I

---

[2] Dr. David Baker and Natacha Keramidas, "The psychology of hunger", American Psychological Association, October 2013, https://www.apa.org/monitor/2013/10/hunger.

was being ridiculous, I bent down and helped pull him up into his lift chair and cleaned up the smoothie.

After cleaning up the smoothie mess, I flew into my car and speeded a bit. Normally, I would stay overnight when I had to drive this far, but I needed to be home to take care of Steve that night. I wanted to cry, laugh, and scream all at once. I felt like a film crew was secretly recording me in this hidden-camera-type moment. Do other caregivers go through this? I could feel myself changing. My joy seemed granule now. It was as if I could count the moments of joy in my life as if they were grains of sand, so finite, so minuscule, so minute by minute.

For years, no one rescued me from my role as a full-time, unwilling caregiver. It was me, day in and day out. In all fairness to family and friends, I didn't tell anyone I needed rescuing. I was too ashamed by my perceived weakness. Finally, after Steve was sick and debilitated for about four years, confined to a wheelchair, and requiring round-the-clock care, I started asking a few people to help, and we put together a patchwork of care to manage his needs.

One person was Joanne, the wife of James, who was Jacob and Emily's school bus driver. A sweet, strong lady with a big smile and a Southern accent, she was a fabulous cook. James also pastored a church and did construction in his free time. Since Joanne was a pastor's wife, Steve loved to hear her talk about church and the Bible.

Joanne normally showed up at 7:00 a.m. and stayed until about 10:00 a.m. She was a huge help, beginning the day with crushing and preparing the fifty pills Steve took each day. Most of them were administered through

Chapter 11

his feeding tube, so there was a lot of separating, crushing, mixing, and preparing in the morning.

Once she was done with that, she helped me by doing laundry and picking up around the house. She was a great cook and would prepare Steve's breakfast of choice. Usually this meant some form of scrambled eggs that he nibbled on throughout the day. His doctor wanted him to take nutrition only through the feeding tube, but he loved food too much to be satisfied with just liquid nutrition. He wanted to taste food. I didn't argue; there were too many other things to worry about. It might take him hours to eat them, but he loved eggs.

Joanne was not a trained nurse but had been one of the best caregivers either one of us could have hoped for. We paid her to help care for Steve three hours a day.

Joanne had several people she cleaned houses for each day and had to leave by 10:00 a.m. Once she left, Steve's mom Louise showed up for the afternoon. Though she was eighty years old, she was in great shape and could daily drive the five miles to our house. She administered his medicine through the feeding tube and kept him company during the day.

The Beautiful Destruction of My Life

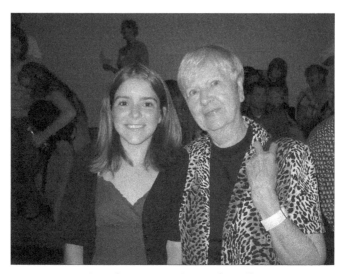

Steve's mom Louise and Emily

I was always afraid of leaving Steve alone even for a short while. We lived in a rural part of the county, and if anyone tried to break into the house, Steve would have been unable to call for help.

Once Jacob and Emily got home from school around 3:00 p.m., Louise left and drove home. The kids watched over Dad until I got home between 5:30 and 6:00 p.m., then I took over his care.

Having to struggle with daycare for my husband was something I never would have dreamed would happen, but we didn't have the funds to hire a home health care worker to care for him. So surrogate family and Joanne were our only solutions. Also, because Steve had a feeding tube, the health care agencies informed me only a registered nurse could provide care, and RNs were expensive.

At times, I felt resentful of being the main caregiver for Steve. Being a caregiver was difficult on sunny days with cloudless skies, even in the best of conditions. On rainy days, well, my patience would reach its limit. When it did, I reminded myself that I was caring for someone who loved me more than any other man would. I was caring for a husband who would do the same for me in a heartbeat and would not complain nearly as much as I did.

Was I flawed? Or just human? Was I ungrateful for all I had? Or just exhausted? Was I deserving of being self-critical? Or lacking in self-compassion?

It's so confusing when your life has been turned topsy-turvy, and after years of working to achieve some stability, you're thrown into a hurricane.

God, what would I do without You to lean on?

As I laid in bed that night, I thought about how compassionate I felt toward Steve most of the time, and for my children, who no longer had a father to take them out for ice cream, teach them to play baseball, or make the money they needed for new clothes.

Then I thought about myself. *Why do I practice compassion for others but not for myself? Don't I deserve the same kindness and forgiveness for not being perfect, for being sometimes grumpy and resentful? I'm not Mother Theresa.* I think, in part, it's a cultural thing. The woman's role is as a caregiver. *So, stop complaining,* I would tell myself. Then I would stop and think. *If I'm not looking out for myself, I'm going to burn out and not do anyone any good.*

I needed to have self-compassion to recharge my batteries and have the emotional energy I needed to care for Steve and my kids. If I attacked myself for getting ornery or feeling that I wasn't doing enough, I would feel too stressed and lash out at my family. Or become depressed, and my kids would have a sick father and depressed mother.

To be a better mom, wife, and caregiver, I needed to make every attempt to be kind toward myself, to not ridicule myself for feeling tired, resentful, unhappy, not feel sorry for myself because my life is so hard. I made a commitment to take care of my mental and physical health as much as I could.

As I had so little time for myself, so I set aside thirty minutes when I got home from work each day for exercise, my only "me" time. I explained to Steve and the kids that this was my one time for myself, and I almost begged them to understand I didn't want to lose it. This was the only non-negotiable thing I did for myself as a caregiver.

Since I have always loved the outdoors, the easiest and cheapest way to release stress and frustration was a daily walk or a short run. As soon as I walked in the door from work, I quickly put on my exercise clothes and tennis shoes and headed down our road before anyone had a chance to stop me. With my earphones in and my favorite music, songs like "Troubadour" by George Strait and "Wide Open Spaces" by the Chicks, I floated down the road and escaped from life.

I would sing these songs out loud as I ran or walked and pretended, I was free and did not have any requirements placed on me to care for anyone else. They would take me to a different time in my life and a better mindset. By the time I made it back home, I was in a better mood and felt I had enough strength to tackle the evening caregiver activities.

Chapter 11

So committed was I to this routine that I went out even in the bitter cold. I remember one time it was so cold it was sleeting. I forced myself to go. I would layer up, put on a hat and gloves, and head out the door. As much as I despised the cold, I despised more skipping my *me* time.

Chapter 12

For years, Steve and I planted a garden. Beginning in early January, we would start making big plans for this beautiful garden. It would be at least an acre of beautifully tilled soil without a single weed. The rows would be evenly spaced. The soil would be so soft and luxurious you could practically sleep on it without a blanket.

Every evening in the summertime, we would walk out to this luxurious garden, collect the fresh, ripe produce in beautiful wicker baskets lined with handmade tea towels, sip on ice-cold homemade lemonade, and return to the Martha Stewart-style kitchen to prepare our fresh bounty.

Seed catalogues would begin to arrive with frenzy. The delivery costs of our catalogues alone paid the salary of at least one mail carrier. The pages turned down and circled, Steve would pick out flowers and plants. Then the ordering would begin, with Steve completely overestimating our abilities to manage a garden.

I dreaded this impending rite of spring. While Steve had visions of something from *Southern Living*©, my idea of raising fresh produce was a small container garden like the one I had planted in the third grade. Needless to say, the yield of the garden usually ended up much closer to my third-grade project. Does that make me a visionary? Still, I put in much work to make our garden bloom.

Once Steve could no longer contribute, gardening, along with twenty-four-hour caregiving, a full-time job, and a cranky, unwilling daughter was a garden of disaster, adding unwanted extra work for Jacob, Emily, and me.

Emily hated gardening. "Mom, my legs are red. I think I am allergic to the dirt," Emily would say.

"No, my dear, you are allergic to work," I said with a sarcastic smile. "Your legs are red because you are lying in the dirt, playing." At this, she tsked and snarled and retreated to her room where no plants existed.

My journey as a caregiver matched our plans for a garden. I started full of energy and enthusiasm, planned how we would survive this disease, read every article on how to be a caregiver, dreamed about where we grow in life as husband and wife, and maybe grandparents someday, and how our garden of life might bloom.

I soon learned my plans are not His plans, but His plans are always better than mine. I learned that the soil we were planted in—our family and friends—would erode in places we didn't expect. I learned that weeds (unhelpful people) would need to be plucked out. I learned that some flowers (friends and family) were only meant for a season and would diminish and disappear as soon as it became cold and hard.

Disease divides friends and family into those strong enough to withstand the disease process and those who aren't. The more Steve's disease progressed, leaving him unable to move and communicate, visitors who hadn't seen him for a while were shocked at what he had become or how badly he looked. Several of Steve's closest friends and family members no longer called or came around.

One day, I bumped into one of his old friends at the grocery store. He pulled me aside.

"I know I don't come around that much anymore. It's just hard for me to see Steve like he is. He's lost so much weight. He looks emaciated. He can't talk. He's in a wheelchair. I want to remember the man he used to be."

I nodded my head. "I know. I understand."

And I did. I, too, wanted to remember the big, smart, interesting man I fell in love with, married, and hoped to spend the rest of my life with. I didn't have that luxury; I had to live with a husband who had gone from 220 to 150 pounds, who could no longer walk, talk, feed himself, or go to the bathroom without assistance.

Instead of getting upset with him, my natural reaction, I accepted his limitations, understanding that he wasn't strong enough to handle our situation and be with us in our pain. Why waste time belaboring the loss? This disease had taught me life is too short to be upset with friends and family for their shortcomings.

The loss of family and friends hit Steve hard and added great, emotional pain to the physical debilitation. He couldn't tell me through words, but I could see it in his eyes. Fortunately, for every friend who caused a small place of erosion or every family member who disappeared when it got tough, God enriched a new place in our garden soil. New friends and additional family members were planted in our lives and grew in ways we never expected, like Joanne, my morning helper. Our church family, my work family, Steve's work family, friends from out of state, and people we met unexpectedly during a meal or hospital stay became our strength and encouragement.

Our church family embraced us in time of need. Dwight was a deacon, and his wife Donna became extremely close to both of us. They had three daughters close to our age but loved us like their own family. In addition to serving as a deacon in the church, they owned a local ice cream stand that was a town favorite.

Dwight and Donna checked on us regularly. More times than I can count, they stepped in to take care of a need or coordinate a resource for us. Steve was partial to the tangerine milkshakes they sold at the ice cream stand. To spoil Steve, they would drop off a box of milkshakes regularly to keep in the freezer. More importantly, they were there to listen, give a hug, and offer advice anytime we needed it.

One day at our church, we were introduced to the new pastor Jeff, who resembled Robert DeNiro, and his wife Rachel, a very sweet, friendly, petite woman with a short, silver-colored, pixie-style haircut. Steve and I both felt an instant friendship with them. They were about fifteen years older than we were, but we got along so well.

Chapter 12

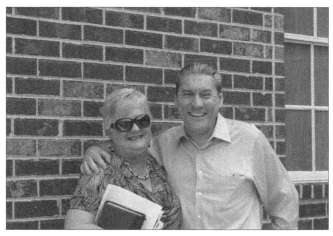

Jeff and Rachel

As the pastor, Jeff liked to joke around. This endeared him to the kids at the church who really liked him.

Rachel would soon become one of my closest friends. We shared a love of shopping at thrift stores and started chatting on the phone every day on my way to work. Possessing a gift for service and loving to cook, she would cook dishes for our family when she could or help me out around the house.

Jeff and Rachel had a daughter about ten years younger than us who was going through a terrible battle with cancer. Their struggles with a deadly disease gave them tremendous empathy for the struggles we daily faced, and around them, we could be a normal couple because they could see beyond the wheelchair and disease. A couple of times we went out to eat with them, as Jeff and Rachel helped me with Steve's wheelchair. It was one of the few times going out to a restaurant was enjoyable, and Steve was happy.

Tommy, Steve's cousin, and his wife Valerie were also a tight part of our inner friendship circle. They went to church with us and lived just down the road, and Tommy came to visit Steve often. Several times, Tommy brought his ATV vehicle and would help Steve get in and take him for a ride around just to see the outdoors.

Thankfully, their house was wheelchair-accessible, and they would invite us to their house for dinner. They had two boys, Matthew and Jeffrey, who were close in age to Jacob and Emily. Hanging out with their cousins was some of the few times that Jacob and Emily could be with kids their age and escape from Dad's wheelchair and disease.

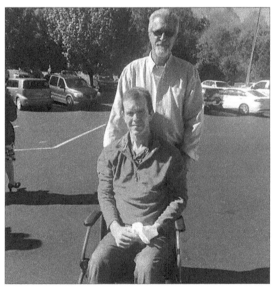

Steve and Tommy

Chapter 13

Amid Steve's disease and my journey in caregiving, I developed an unlikely friendship. Kim was a new friend to me who offered to regularly help us out. I never suspected I would become eternally grateful for Steve's high-school sweetheart.

I had been introduced to her about eighteen years before when Steve and I went to one of his class reunions. While she was friendly and I, in turn, pleasant to her, something in me didn't like her. Why should I? She was my husband's former girlfriend, and we had the same name.

They had dated for five years. She was beautiful with magical, long, blond, wavy hair, a slender and fit figure, kind smile, wide green eyes, and Southern charm like it was dripping in melted butter and warm pancake syrup. I was sick to my stomach thinking about how sweet she was.

I was jealous—of course. I lacked her Southern charm. No way could all that charm be genuine. She was trying to impress me; I was sure of it. She wanted to make me jealous.

To make matters worse, Steve's family had always talked affectionately about her. Yes, even thirty years later, they loved her. His mom and dad never failed to let me know how sweet they thought Kim was and that she still came to visit the family. Really? What was this girl's motive? Why on earth would you visit your ex-childhood sweetheart's family many years later unless you had an ulterior motive?

I knew she was a wolf in sheep's clothing. Fortunately, while Steve was still in the Navy, we lived out of state, so the chance of our paths crossing again anytime soon was highly unlikely.

Or so I thought.

Years after Steve left the Navy, we met again at her church after moving back to his hometown. Great, now on top of her being beautiful and having a great personality, she was also an active member of her church and had everyone fooled that she was Sister Super Christian. It was getting harder not to like her. I was trying my best to uncover her faults, but as hard as I tried, I couldn't figure out a reason to not like her.

Then one day, I was reading in our local newspaper a feature story about her donating a kidney to one of her family members. Good grief! "Miss Magical Hair, is there anything you can't do?" Ah, maybe that's a reason to not like her. She's too perfect. Something must be wrong with her.

It got worse. On top of all her fantastic characteristics, it seemed God had blessed her with a servant's heart. As Steve's MSA progressed, she made several attempts to befriend me and offer help.

About four years in, Steve's MSA continued to progress to a point where digestion slowed to a crawl. Any food

Chapter 13

he could consume was extremely slow to pass through his intestines and would often stall there. This caused him to suffer a bowel obstruction in addition to extreme constipation, and he had been hospitalized multiple times. One time, he was hospitalized for ten days. He returned home bedridden with a feeding tube and was temporarily placed on TPN (Total Parenteral Nutrition), a method of feeding through an IV that bypasses the gastrointestinal tract.

The return home was excruciating on me. Overnight we went from round-the-clock nursing care in the progressive care unit to just me. I was now responsible for every aspect of daily living, including maintaining the TPN and flushing the IV lines every day. This meant after I got myself up and dressed each day, I had to help Steve move over or reposition him in the bed, change the bed sheets, empty his foley catheter, brush his teeth, get the remote control for the TV, reposition him again in the bed, get him dressed, wash his face, and make sure he had something to drink to keep his mouth moist.

He hated being stuck in our bedroom on the backside of the house, but we didn't have a choice in the matter. The hospital offered to arrange a hospital bed for Steve that would have been helpful, but in our tiny house, there was no room for one. We would have had to move the couch to the front porch if we brought a hospital bed in. Instead, we chose to make do in our small bedroom. Jacob helped me bring in a chair, so if Steve had company, they could sit down and talk to him instead of just standing and looking at Steve in the bed.

Kim called shortly after we got home and offered to bring dinner to us. Steve couldn't eat, but the kids and I sure could. I was too tired to tell her no and, reluctantly, I accepted her kindness.

She showed up toting her homemade goodness. I anticipated she would have picked up some form of carryout for us. Nope. She showed up with an actual picnic basket straight out of the Martha Stewart collection full of homemade Chinese broccoli and chicken, complete with rice and eggrolls. I was impressed and secretly jealous that she had time to cook a meal.

Her blond, wavy hair was perfect in a low, messy bun and perfectly done makeup to look natural, with a hint of shimmer on her lips; she was beautifully dressed in her black Capri workout pants, neon-colored name-brand athletic shirt, and running shoes. Ugh. She was even perfect when she worked out.

I, on the other hand, looked and felt the worst I had in years. The time in the hospital and now serving as an unpaid and untrained nurse was wearing on me. My hair was an uncombed mess, wrapped up with a ponytail to some version of a messy bun—very messy bun, nothing like her perfectly coiffed hair. The house was filthy, cluttered, and full of medical supplies. I wore the same sweats and T-shirt I slept in.

It was one of those days where you don't want to see anyone. Wow, what luck do I have? On one of the worst days of my life, the prom queen was coming over. I don't know if guys care what they look like in front of other guys, but girls always do. It doesn't matter if we have been shipwrecked on a deserted island. We still want to look our best if anyone visits us on that deserted island.

Chapter 13

I hated to admit it, but the food was really good. It was all homemade, not the store-bought goodness that I usually default to. She was starting to get to me. There was a remote chance she might be genuinely doing this out of the goodness of her heart. Notice I said "remote chance" because I still didn't trust her. She was far too beautiful and kind to trust. That stuff doesn't come naturally, at least in my experience.

Over the next year, Steve recovered enough to where he had the strength to come off the TPN and get out of bed and back up into the wheelchair. This allowed him to venture back to the living room, but improvements were meager. Each hospital stay seemed to wear him down further, and my role as caregiver was now like trying to take care of a giant forty-eight-year-old baby, as he was unable to do anything on his own. I had to dress him, feed him, change him, take him to the bathroom, and bathe him.

Unable to communicate in barely any intelligible way, he mainly whispered and tried to mouth words, frustrating him tremendously. I could tell when he wanted me to know something but couldn't get his vocal cords to work or the words to form on his lips. He would tense up and glare his eyes at me as if he was mad. My heart ached for the frustration he was feeling.

As the year went on, Kim's kindness and thoughtfulness continued to wear me down. She sent cards of encouragement and friendship. She offered to help clean my house. I, of course, viewed this as her sending me a subtle hint that my house was messy. God had a greater plan here that I didn't see. Slowly over the year, we started to develop a friendship.

Steve had now been sick for about five years. When Kim entered our lives, he could not eat enough to sustain himself and required daily feeding through his feeding tube, though he loved the idea of food and often wanted us to leave it in his mouth. He could barely drink much on his own, swallowing was difficult, and his doctors often discouraged him from eating or drinking anything. His breathing would sometimes be labored as well.

One day, Kim invited me to go hiking. Steve encouraged me to go, and I lined up a friend to stay with Steve for the day. He knew how much I struggled with caregiving. He worried, though, that I wouldn't keep up with her. "Kim is a world-class hiker," he informed me by slowly typing a message to me on his laptop. Apparently, she had convinced everyone she scaled the likes of Mount Everest on a regular basis.

"I'm going hiking just to prove I can," I said. "I don't care if it kills me." I don't know why; I am not competitive.

I prepared for our hiking adventure as a complete novice. Not having fancy hiking clothes or gear, I wore a pair of drawstring khaki pants and an old windbreaker I picked up at Goodwill for this occasion. I pulled my hair up and donned my headband. None of my attire really matched, but I didn't care. I figured make-up and jewelry would be of no use. After all, we would be hiking in the wilderness and wouldn't see anyone.

Chapter 13

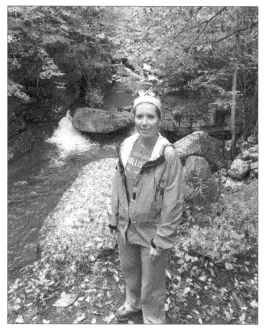

Me first time hiking

Wouldn't you know it? Kim showed up dressed to kill in her name-brand fancy hiking gear, appropriate hiking boots, magical hair perfectly coiffed, air-brushed make-up, and selfie stick in tow. This should have been my first red flag. I didn't know hiking meant the equivalent of a wilderness photo shoot.

I survived the hike, the wilderness photo shoot, and learned some valuable lessons that day. She really was a world-class hiker, and we took some fun pictures of our adventure. Hmmm. I truly had a best friend in the works.

Since meeting Kim, I have learned there's little she can't do. Kim is adventurous. For some reason, part of her adventure seemed to be to become my best friend. I had no idea why. I was no prize as a friend. I was worn-to-the-bone tired from caregiving and had little if any free time to do things. I had nothing exciting to share about my life other than I was tired and worn-out. All I talked about was medical procedures. I had little to offer in return in the friendship. Still, she persisted.

One day, she and I were talking outside on my front porch about some of the struggles we were both facing in life. Steve was sitting in his chair in the living room within my sight. It was becoming nice to have a friend who wanted to spend time with me and didn't mind helping me with Steve's care. By this time, we had been friends for about a year. Her husband of twenty-five years, who was only in his early fifties, ironically had been diagnosed with Parkinson's disease. As MSA and Parkinson's shared some similar characteristics, we realized we shared some similar struggles. Not only had she been the first person to reach out to me, but she was also capable of understanding the nightmare I was going through as a caregiver.

As she pulled out of the driveway, I realized something. I may, possibly, just might almost have a genuine friendship with this girl who was Steve's high-school sweetheart first; all things God had in mind when giving me the unlikely strength of her friendship. God had a perfect plan between the two of us. This was the stuff of which movies are made.

Chapter 13

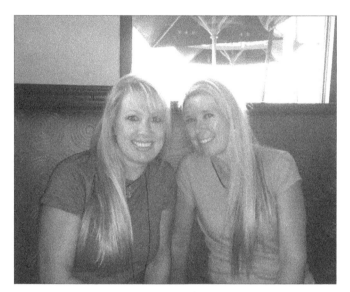

Kim and I

Chapter 14

I woke up and looked around, realizing we were at the stage in this dreadful disease where everything was messy. There was no time to clean up anything in my life that was messy: my house, clothes, hair, finances, parenting, and relationships. In our little 1,000-square-foot home, we had four people, one very large, motorized wheelchair, and three Chihuahuas trying to find space.

It seemed like every inch of available wall space in the hallways was strategically lined with wire shelves that I purchased at the local home improvement store. Every time I ran out of space to store the pots and pans, groceries, and boxes of ongoing medical supplies, I would add a new shelf. I loved to watch home-decorating shows and read articles on Pinterest of the best new way to create a farmhouse look. None of my wire shelves have any resemblance of farmhouse.

Caregiving had sucked the life out of my bones, and it stole our marriage. Somewhere in the last couple of years, we transitioned from husband and wife to nurse and patient. I don't know when it happened. It would have been easier if it happened overnight, and I could identify this line in the sand. Instead, it had happened gradually over the last couple of years. I didn't love him any less, and I don't think of him any less; it was just that our roles in our marriage were different.

I missed being able to talk with Steve. With every ounce of me, I missed having a conversation with him. He was right next to me, but we couldn't have a conversation. There were no words that came out of his mouth, just gasps and whispers. He struggled and craned his neck in a contortion due to the dystonia, which would cause his muscles to spasm and is a condition that has gradually come on due to the high amount of Carbidopa Levodopa Steve was taking to manage the symptoms of his Multiple System Atrophy.

His eyes would glare at me almost as if he was in pain. He was not in physical pain, but I knew he was in emotional pain, the pain of not being able to speak or talk at all. I missed being able to tell him about my day and asking him about his day. I missed being able to ask him his opinion on the world, religion, politics, the kids, finances, and even celebrity gossip. It's pointless to ask.

This created a gap between us we didn't know how to fix. I didn't want to put him through the pain of trying to talk, as well as the physical and emotional pain of me trying to listen. I had to get so close that I pressed my ear close to his mouth to understand the gasps. It took forever and was probably mere minutes, but it felt like hours standing over his wheelchair with my ear to his mouth, trying to figure out what he was saying. I would have never guessed that this was one of the things I missed the most with this dreaded disease.

Chapter 14

We used to text each other throughout our workday. Now I could no longer text "I love you" during the day. He still had his cellphone, but it didn't serve a purpose anymore. He was unable to use his hands on the keys of the phone. When I texted him, someone could help him read it, but someone else had to pick his phone up and respond for him. It was no longer an intimate text between us. I couldn't call him during my day to see how his day was going. It was a mess, and my life seemed like it was turning into a big mess one piece at a time.

Chapter 15

*Y*ou ever have one of those years when you look back and think, *Wow, that was a great year?* Even in the midst of a terminal illness, we had one of those years.

It began on January 1, 2015. Steve was at a mild plateau. His disease hadn't progressed in almost a year. He had not been hospitalized in a year. He was still wheelchair-bound and completely unable to do anything on his own, but we were happy. We were hopeful it would stay that way.

Our life dream had always been to build a house on our property. We were living in a tiny house completely inaccessible for Steve's wheelchair. The walls and doorways were scarred with wheelchair marks everywhere. With life in such a crazy state and regular hospital stays, we had put off that dream, never knowing whether he would live or die.

On New Year's Eve, Jacob, Emily, and I had stayed up until midnight to celebrate the New Year. I was thankful they didn't have plans to spend the New Year with any friends. We did our usual family tradition of watching

Dick Clark's New Year's Rocking Eve, making some finger foods, and watching the ball drop at midnight.

I had helped Steve get into bed around 10:00 p.m. He could not transfer on his own but could tense his muscles enough so that I could pivot him and get him into bed on my own. I could have gone to sleep at 10:00, but I felt it wasn't fair to Jacob and Emily to ring in the New Year on their own because I was too tired. I always made a wish for the New Year and prayed for the possibilities—the possibility of healing for Steve and a way for our lives to be easier.

When Steve woke up on New Year's Day, he seemed to have a fresh approach. He had a bit of a smile on his face. Steve never complained to me about his disease. Never once during the entire time he was diagnosed with MSA did he say, "Why me?" or that he was mad. He knew God had a plan for his life and never questioned that plan.

Like him, I never complained to him about being his caregiver. It wasn't fair; he didn't ask to be sick. He wasn't doing this on purpose. He never deserved to be sick. Words have power, and I was careful not to ever share my frustration with caregiving to him. He knew I was tired, but I never got angry with him.

Through slow whispers, he told me he was ready to build the house we had always dreamed of on our property. I was shocked. How on earth was I going to make the decisions needed to build a house in addition to caring for Steve?

Though the idea was crazy, Steve and I had prayed for years to do this. When God answers a prayer, He also provides a way. Steve had saved ideas for years on how

Chapter 15

he wanted a house to be built, what products he wanted, and had researched all the latest trends in accessible home design.

We met with a couple of builders, and in March 2015, signed a contract with a local builder to start. We were able to obtain the financing necessary and started. Fortunately, our builder was fantastic to work with. He was patient with Steve's inability to communicate but still kept him in on the progress.

Most of the decisions went through me, and I would share with Steve what was happening. Unfortunately, once construction began, Steve could only view progress from the car. There was no way to get his wheelchair in the house, and it was way too dangerous.

I took lots of pictures of the progress, and every day we would look at ideas together. Building a house gave Steve a renewed sense of purpose. He couldn't do much, but he could still look up things on the computer. His mind was still active.

During building, we received two more amazing blessings that year: an honor for Steve and a retreat for the family. In the spring, a friend of mine from work nominated Steve for an Honor Air Knoxville flight. The Honor Flight Network is an amazing organization created solely to **honor** America›s veterans for all their sacrifices. They transport heroes to Washington, DC, to visit and reflect on their memorials.

The logistics of flying to Washington DC and visiting memorials would have been a monumental undertaking for me alone. Honor Air Knoxville had it down to a science. They allowed me to accompany Steve because he was unable to communicate very well and required medicine every three hours. This organization runs on multitudes of volunteers and is accompanied by an esteemed team of medical staff volunteering their time from the local hospital.

We boarded an airplane out of Knoxville, Tennessee, and landed a short time later in Washington, DC, to a nostalgic band playing patriotic songs and lots of people greeting the flight and waving American flags. There were even men and women in WWII-era dress, hair appropriately coiffed and swing dancing.

After landing in our nation's capital, the veterans on the flight were quickly ushered to coach buses ready to go. This would not be a normal trip through the capital. The buses were chaperoned and guided through the streets of Washington, DC, by two motorcycle police officers. With their blue lights flashing and sirens going, they stopped traffic so the coaches could drive unobstructed and quickly guided the veterans straight to their memorials.

We visited four memorials that day. At noon, we stopped for a break and sat in the chilly air at the Air Force Memorial to eat sandwiches from boxed lunches. I was delighted to see a smile spread across Steve's face the entire day. His service in the Navy had meant a lot to him, and this was a great way for him to relive some of that.

Chapter 15

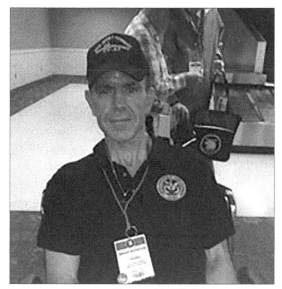

Steve Honor Air Flight

The flight returned to Knoxville about 8:00 p.m. that evening to a welcome home no one expected. The entire corridor of the airport was lined with hundreds of well-wishers to thank the veterans and show appreciation for their military service. Patriotic songs played in the background. Families held up thank-you signs. Boy Scouts in uniform shook hands. At the end, Jacob and Emily greeted Steve, having been brought by some of our church friends, who drove the hour to the airport so they could see Dad come off the plane.

Still excited from the Honor Air trip, we were blessed again upon learning that our family had been chosen to receive an all-expenses-paid weekend retreat from an organization called Inheritance of Hope (IOH). To me, it was as if we had won the lottery!

This wonderful nonprofit organization was created by Deric and Kristen Milligan to inspire hope in young families facing the loss of a parent due to a terminal illness. Unfortunately, we met their qualifications. Betsy from IOH called to invite us to attend a retreat in Orlando, Florida, on Memorial Day weekend.

I packed up the wheelchair van and drove our family the 600-mile trek to Orlando. Though the trip was long and difficult, as expected, we were all filled with excitement, imagining what this surprise retreat might be like. Along the way, Betsy had called me to ask how soon we would be arriving at the hotel. She wanted regular updates to see when we would be there.

I dreaded the arrival at the hotel. There would be all the luggage to unload. Jacob and Emily would be antsy since they had been stuck in the van. Steve would be tired and ready to get out or at least lie down and stretch his legs on the bed. I would have to stand in line to check in and figure out how to get our luggage up to the room. Never mind that I was the one doing all the driving.

What a shock when we pulled into the hotel! A team of volunteers from IOH met us at the entrance, excited and clapping. They immediately opened the doors of the van and unloaded all the luggage. I didn't know what to say. My only job once they unloaded Steve and the van was to go park the van a short distance away. They would have done that too if I wanted them to!

Once I got back inside the hotel, Betsy greeted me with a set of keys to our hotel room. To my surprise, they had already taken Steve, the kids, and all our luggage to the room. Once in the room, this wonderful organization and several caring volunteers even had cookies, T-shirts, and welcome notes waiting for us.

We checked into the hotel Saturday night and started our retreat with a group dinner. It was so refreshing to be around other families facing the loss of a parent. I got a chance to meet other caregivers, and, most importantly, Jacob and Emily could meet kids going through some of the same feelings they were going through. They got to be normal kids for the first time in years.

After dinner, all the families had an opportunity for a personal family photo session with Mickey Mouse. Emily connected right away with a couple of teenagers named MaryAnn and Michael. They came up to our hotel room later in the evening to get Emily, and they all went back to a spot in the lobby to eat popcorn and talk. I was so happy Emily had found some friends to connect with. Jacob was more reserved and was just happy to be on a vacation. He enjoyed his first night at the hotel playing his handheld video games.

The Beautiful Destruction of My Life

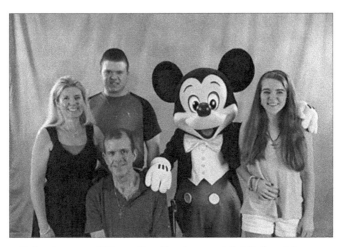

Inheritance of Hope family photo with Mickey Mouse

Sunday morning would begin with counseling sessions for each of us and then an afternoon trip to Disney World for the group.

While giving Steve a shower, I noticed his feeding tube lying on the floor of the shower. This had never happened before. His doctor had told me previously that if his feeding tube ever came out, it would need to be replaced within a few hours. The opening can close quickly, so we didn't have much time to find a specialist. Sunday morning in a different state, the only option was a trip to the emergency room. We hadn't even been on our retreat twenty-four hours, and we were already headed to the ER. Thankfully, the volunteers from IOH immediately took action and chaperoned Emily and Jacob so they could go to Disney World. Unfortunately, when living with a terminal disease, you never know when it is going to rear its ugly head and ruin your plans.

Chapter 15

We ended up spending six hours in the ER that Sunday before the medical team could replace his feeding tube with another one. However, they didn't have an adult feeding tube, only a pediatric feeding tube. It would work temporarily until we could make it back to Steve's doctor in Tennessee. The doctor inserted the new feeding tube, and we headed back to the hotel. Deric, the CEO of IOH, escorted us from the hotel to Disney World to meet up with Jacob and Emily and at least enjoy a few hours as a family at Disney World. It truly was magical.

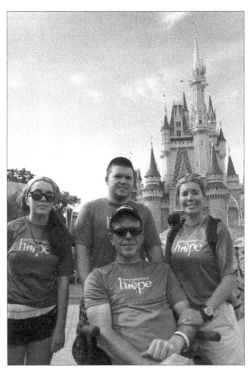

Inheritance of Hope Retreat family photo at Disney World

The rest of the weekend with IOH was amazing. We all received counseling each day, but not the traditional counseling. I got to sit in a room with other caregivers and talk about what it was like to be a caregiver. It was an awesome feeling to find out others were feeling the exact same way: stressed, tired, angry, sad, disappointed, scared, and lonely. That is what it felt like to be a caregiver.

Jacob and Emily's counseling allowed them to express feelings in ways that were helpful to them as teenagers. IOH had experienced, trained professionals on site to help kids of all ages work through their grief and fears. They played games, laughed, and even made collages from pictures in old magazines of how they saw their lives. They had the freedom to talk about what each picture meant to them and how they felt about it.

On Monday night, Steve and I had the luxury of a date night arranged by IOH. They made plans for Jacob and Emily to go out with the other teenagers for pizza and games.

Before our date, Steve and I had the opportunity to make a legacy video—a message to Jacob and Emily that would live on when we would no longer be altogether as a family. This was perhaps the hardest thing either of us had ever done.

We were in a quiet room in the hotel with Betsy from IOH guiding us through some questions. Mostly we were talking directly to Jacob and Emily for them to view after Steve's death.

Steve and I shared the story of how we met and married. Much of the time, I interpreted what Steve was trying to share about how much he loved both and was

Chapter 15

proud of them. When he tried to talk, it was very difficult to push air through his vocal cords, so sounds were about a whisper.

In addition, the MSA had progressed to a point where he had acute dystonia, in which a person's muscles contract uncontrollably. When he tried to talk, his body seemed to contort in painful positions that he couldn't control. In the end, both Steve and I cried painful tears, knowing the impact of this video, and realizing they would not watch it until Steve had passed away.

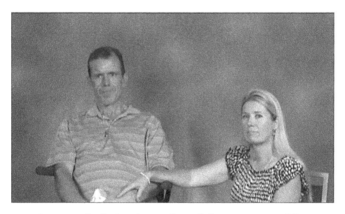

Steve and I being interviewed for a Legacy Video

After the video, Steve and I went by ourselves to a Japanese hibachi-style restaurant. Since this was the first real date night we had in about six years, I had put a bit of extra effort into dressing up. I wore a black cotton mini skirt that fell just above my knee, sandals with a little bit of silver glitter, and a black-and-white, dressy, short-sleeved top. I even wore my favorite silver hoop earrings.

I dressed Steve in a blue and salmon-colored, short-sleeved cotton polo shirt and khaki shorts, and I applied my favorite cologne on him and put on his slip-on loafers. It is a bit strange to have to dress my date, push his wheelchair down to the van, load him in the van, and then drive us to the restaurant, but that was our reality.

We enjoyed a nice time together since we were rarely alone and never on a date. Steve ate a little bit. With a feeding tube, he wasn't supposed to be eating much at this point but loved the taste of food. He could still chew small bites of food, but it took him forever to get any food down.

Jacob and Emily returned full of smiles from their night out. Emily had been with Dianna and MaryAnn and some other kids from IOH whom she had connected with. They quickly left Emily's room to find a hiding spot in the lobby to talk like normal teenage girls do. Normally, I would have been concerned about her going to the lobby by herself, but the hotel was full of IOH staff and volunteers and plenty of security to chaperone. I wanted to give Emily the freedom to be as normal as possible, even if just for a weekend.

Tuesday was time to say our goodbyes. We had a closing ceremony in the morning with our new IOH family. It was more than bittersweet, though, because Steve had started feeling sick. I knew what was happening. He had several bowel obstructions in the past and had been hospitalized multiple times for them. My worst fear of him getting sick in another state was likely coming true. Still, we had already decided to stay one more night in Orlando to enjoy Florida a bit more before heading back to Tennessee on Wednesday, and we did.

Chapter 15

Late Tuesday night, Steve started vomiting. As much as I didn't want to have to take him to the hospital, I knew I had to, and we headed to Dr. Phillips Hospital in Orlando. After assessing Steve in the ER and determining he had a fever, they admitted him. Jacob and Emily had stayed behind at the hotel. Jacob was nineteen, and Emily was seventeen, so they were fine in the hotel overnight.

I went back to the hotel in the morning. We were scheduled to check out that day, but I had no idea what to do. I went to the front desk, talked to the manager, and explained my situation. They allowed us to extend our stay for a couple of days to allow me time to figure out what to do in the hope that Steve would be ready to go home by then.

Thursday came, and Steve's condition was not improving. At one point, his blood pressure dropped drastically, and he was barely conscious. He did have an obstruction in his intestine, but it was not completely blocked. They also found he had two large stones in one of his kidneys: one twenty-one millimeters and the other eight millimeters. He had been on an intermittent catheter for years, so this didn't tremendously surprise us. However, it didn't appear to be causing any problems.

On Thursday night, I called our families. I hated asking for help, but I needed to find a way to either get someone to help Jacob and Emily stay in Orlando or have someone from Tennessee come and pick them up. I didn't think they were prepared to fly on their own, and I didn't think Steve would be up for the drive back home once we got out of the hospital.

Fortunately, Steve's cousin Tommy offered to fly to Orlando the next day and drive our van back to Tennessee with Jacob and Emily and most of our luggage. Tommy is a truck driver and tall, probably about six-foot-two, with dark, thick wavy hair, a friendly smile, and a strong Southern accent.

He and his son Jeffrey arrived at the airport in Orlando on Friday. I drove out to pick them up and bring them back to the hospital to check in on Steve. I was so thankful to see a family member and have help making decisions.

That evening, I took Tommy and Jeffery back to stay in our room at the hotel. Thankfully, our room had two double beds and a pullout sofa bed. There was plenty of room for Tommy, Jeffrey, Jacob, and Emily to all stay in the room. I stayed at the hospital with Steve.

They spent all Saturday at the hospital with Steve. Fortunately, he was in a fairly large hospital room that even had a couch. Tommy helped me load up the van and luggage and left Orlando late Saturday night, heading the 600-plus miles back to Tennessee with Jacob and Emily. I had Tommy take Steve's wheelchair home in the van since I didn't think I would need it. At that point, I knew we couldn't drive and figured we would fly home. In my haste, I didn't think we would need a wheelchair.

This left me at the hospital with no vehicle or idea how we were going to get home. Nor did I have any idea how long Steve would be hospitalized.

By the following Tuesday, Steve had now been hospitalized for a week, and the blockage started to improve enough that we could consider making the trip back home. I found a flight departing Orlando on Thursday afternoon

Chapter 15

we could take. Tuesday night, I started making sure I had everything in order for Steve to be discharged on Wednesday, when, to my dismay, I realized I had packed Steve's wallet inadvertently in the van with many of his things. Steve no longer carried his wallet; I always did, and somehow I had it in a bag that I had packed. I made some panicked phone calls to my friend Donna back at home and had to arrange for Jacob to take Steve's wallet to her so she could overnight it to the hotel for me. The amount of precise timing that went into this was scary. The wallet had to be delivered via overnight package to the hotel by 10:30 a.m. the next morning for us to make the 11:00 a.m. shuttle to the airport and get on the flight.

On Wednesday, the hospital discharged Steve, and I called a cab to take us to a hotel right near the airport. I had called ahead, and the hotel told me they would have a shuttle to get us to the airport. There was only one slight problem I hadn't counted on: without Steve's wheelchair, I had no transport to the hotel. I knew the airport would have a wheelchair, but I didn't have a plan for the hotel.

The hotel assured me they had a wheelchair we could use. However, when we arrived, it was clear no one had used the wheelchair in many years. It didn't have the leg rests on the bottom to put your feet on and barely rolled, but it was enough to get Steve up to the room. From there, I used the small task chair in front of the desk that was on wheels to get him into the bathroom and into bed.

The next morning, I was so determined to get out of Orlando and get home I pushed that feebly wheelchair with no leg rests as hard as I could to the elevator and slung our bags over my shoulder to get him downstairs and to the shuttle. Once on the shuttle, we could request a Skycap at the airport with a wheelchair.

I was ever so thankful to get on an airplane and leave Orlando. Our dream four- day family retreat had turned into a ten-day nightmare, where I wasn't even sure we would ever leave Orlando! On the plane ride home, Steve was a little woozy. His blood pressure seemed to go down a bit, and I was afraid he might pass out. To make sure he didn't eliminate our chance to get home, I prodded him the whole way home to stay awake. I am not sure if I threatened or warned him that I was getting out of Orlando with or without him. Thankfully, he made it to Chattanooga awake.

Our return home from the hospital in Orlando was short-lived. We flew into Chattanooga on a Wednesday afternoon. By Thursday morning, Steve was back in a hospital in Knoxville, having a new feeding tube placed in. The feeding tube was the thing that got this whole crazy trip in Orlando started. That darn feeding tube that kept him alive and during this trip seemed to almost kill him and me.

Chapter 16

While leaving a doctor's appointment with Steve, we were in a waiting room the size of a large elevator. As I tried to open the door to leave and go backward through it, about ten people in the waiting room just sat and watched. I guess they were busy with their routines of staring blankly at their cellphones, engrossed in the latest very important pet video or picture of someone's family reunion. I took one hand and pushed open the door, then contorted my hip in a weird position while I dragged Steve's chair backward through the threshold. Someone looked up at me, as if to say, "Oh, I didn't see you there ten feet in front of me struggling." I retorted with a sarcastic "No worries; I am good" as I glared and struggled out of the doorway with Steve and his wheelchair. I am regularly surprised at the insensitivity many people have to the disabled community and wheelchairs. I really don't think it is intentional. I am going to chalk it up to a routine.

Caregiving had become a routine for me every day too. I was not happy about it, but there was no point in being upset or angry about it, no point in being angry about how much of my life had been destroyed by caregiving.

It simply was what my life had become at that point. I was essentially responsible for handling every aspect of daily living for my husband. The sadness from this routine was overwhelming to me. It was like a heavy weight I couldn't put down. I carried it everywhere with me. As overwhelming as the sadness was to me, I could tell others around me felt more sadness for the situation. It was a type of sadness that came from being unable to help.

I promised Steve early in his diagnosis that I would never put him in a nursing care facility. "Of course, I won't put you in a nursing home. Don't be silly." I remembered saying to him, "I can handle taking care of you." At the time, I made the promise, I had no idea what that promise meant. Years of intensive caregiving without a break have changed my perspective. I wish he would have given me permission to take a break, permission even for respite care. Several times at doctor's appointments, they would suggest hospice to Steve. He refused to hear of it, and I agreed with him. I hadn't taken the time to really understand what hospice meant.

Medical professionals don't always do a good job of explaining it either. It was just a tool they offered to you. I thought it meant you were dying, and they would offer medications to make the dying process easier and less painful. I wish I had learned about hospice much sooner. Eventually Steve did decide to enter hospice about five weeks before he passed away. I wish I had given it the credit that this wonderful blessing to the dying and their family deserves.

I wanted a break so badly. I was hoping for someone, anyone, to spend the night with Steve. I would have even

Chapter 16

been willing to sleep in the spare room just so I could get a good night's sleep. It was my fault I probably wouldn't have accepted the help if it was offered. That would have meant I wasn't as strong as I thought I should be.

Sometimes during our daily routine of me getting him out of bed and putting his T-shirt on, I was sad. I looked at this frail man with a feeding tube sticking out of his thin stomach and wonder how we got there. What happened to the tall, rugged military man I married nearly twenty-eight years before? How had this disease taken so much of him and our lives away?

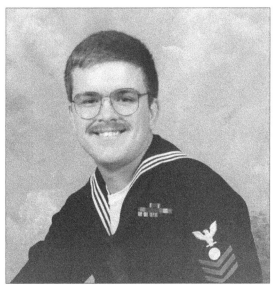

Steve in the early days of our marriage

I would sit back and look at him. Sometimes he didn't know I was watching him. I was hoping to see a glimmer of the Steve I used to know. As I finished getting him dressed, I put on his cologne. The cologne wasn't really for him; it was for me. The scent reminded me of a time gone by, the man he used to be.

Caregiving had taken the life out of me. I felt like an invisible person, and it was hard to figure out where the disease ended, and my life began. The two were so intertwined. Sometimes while I was going through the motions of catheterizing Steve or giving him a shower in this ridiculously small shower stall not meant for two people, I'd mumble to myself how much I hate this life. I would never speak these words out loud. If I said them out loud, I was afraid God would hear them.

I just wanted to be a normal person again.

Chapter 17

Steve was now five years into his official diagnosis of MSA. He was entirely dependent on me for care. He needed me from the minute he woke up until the minute he went to sleep and then some. I no longer lived for one person; I was one person living life for two people.

I provided every aspect of his daily living for him. I transferred him out of the bed and into the wheelchair. I dressed him. I helped him on the toilet, gave him a daily enema, wiped him after he went to the bathroom, and bathed him. It was too cumbersome to take him to the barber, so I started cutting his hair about every other week, as well as put his deodorant on and sprayed cologne on his neck. I fed him, administered his feeding tube supplements, changed the sheets, and administered his medicines.

I drove the car, let the dog out, made the phone calls, went to work, talked to all of the family and friends checking on him, and paid the bills. I was husband and wife. I was Mom and Dad. I was exhausted!

Every day of caregiving depleted me. One particular day, after only four to five hours of sleep, I felt I couldn't go on. The day wasn't worse than any other. Nothing traumatic had happened. I just reached the end of my rope. I could no longer cope with never-ending caregiving with no rest. I cried all the way to work.

To cope and tolerate the constant pressure of my life as a caregiver of having every free minute of my day consumed with caring for another person, I slipped my feelings into little boxes in my mind. If the feeling was inappropriate, like hating being a caregiver, I closed the box in my mind and refused to open it. This technique worked well. Some days, the feelings built up, and the mental box burst open. That day was one of those days.

Here's how I remember it.

I opened a Pandora's box of feelings. I was searching for something and knew it had to be in there. I was sure I put those feeling back in the box for use for later. Surely, I hadn't lost it. I know it had to be there. I would dig and dig.

The feeling box is huge. It is full of darkness and what appears to be a mire of quicksand. If I was not careful, I could sink in this box and never be found again. Some of the feelings were so buried and forbidden they were likely illegal in all but a few shady, third-world countries. There were so many feelings in there. I didn't even know some of them existed in life.

I grabbed onto *miserable*. That wasn't the one I was looking for, but it was available. Why on earth would I want to pull this one out? I had plenty of miserable feelings already. I put *miserable* back at the bottom of the box. Hopefully, it would stay there. The feeling box was cold and dark.

Wait. Here it is. Oops. Wrong again. This was *anger*. Clearly, I didn't want to get any more feelings of anger.

Chapter 17

I was overloaded with feelings of anger and at the most inopportune times. Anger came out when we were running late to a doctor's appointment, and I was the one who had to do everything. I had to get him dressed. Do you know what it was like getting an adult man dressed? Let's just say Levi jeans were not made to be easily slipped into when your legs were paralyzed and the person getting the pants on was half your size!

Wait, I didn't finish all the reasons I was angry. Getting dressed was only a tiny percentage of the battle. There was the bathroom routine: the catheter to prepare and administer, the daily enemas, and then giving him a shower.

There were the medicines to prepare and pack. I counted out the pills, put them in the plastic pill bag, crushed them, and then carefully mixed them in with water and drew them into the syringe. I labeled everything to make sure I gave them at exactly the right time. With more than fifty pills a day, I was now a pharmacist assistant.

There was getting the wheelchair to the van. I would follow him to the van and open the door carefully, so the ramp landed in just the right spot. Once the wheelchair was up into the van, I would get out the four tie-downs to make sure the wheelchair didn't move while we were driving, even though it weighed 250 pounds. I would then finagle my way around the bottom of the wheelchair and ratchet down the tie-downs. I never mastered the ratchet straps for hauling the tractor on his trailer when we were farming, and I had no additional skills to ratchet down a wheelchair.

I was tired just thinking about the memory of it all. I didn't have a right to this feeling. What did I have to be angry about? I wasn't the one who was sick. I wasn't the one in a wheelchair. I wasn't the one having to eat through a feeding tube. I wasn't the one who had lost my voice. I was just the one cleaning up the aftermath of what sickness does to a body, relationship, and family. I had the better part out of this whole deal. Still, I held tight to anger and didn't want to let it go.

Anger was the second step in the grieving process. First was denial. Been there. Done that. Denial was not even in the box. I was grieving for my lost husband, lost dreams, and lost life. I had the right to be angry.

I kept searching. *Tired.* Yep. That was a feeling I owned. It almost jumped into my arms. The kind of tired where your whole body was worn to the bone. I had a legitimate right to this feeling. I was sleeping a total of four to five hours most nights. I never slept an entire night; this had been going on for years. I wasn't meant to keep up this pace of caregiving on this small amount of sleep.

"You can sleep when you die" someone told me as a joke. This was no joking matter. I literally felt I would die if I didn't get sleep and rest from this non-stop onslaught of caregiving.

I had a mission. I need to find a feeling I had lost. I desperately wanted this one back. What was it? Where was it? Instead, I found *lonely*. I felt like the only person in the Western Hemisphere with that feeling. I was a horrible person for having these feelings and wasn't entitled to them. *Lonely* isolated me from everyone. No

Chapter 17

one understood what I was going through as a caregiver. *Lonely* told me there wasn't one person out there who understood.

   My friends and family didn't understand what I was going through. I didn't blame them. They'd never been through this. Sure, a few people told me they helped care for their mom or dad for a few months, but I don't know anyone who had done this for years on end. Only a couple of friends knew what caregiving really meant, like Kim.

   For those who didn't, I didn't try to explain. For one, I wanted to protect Steve's privacy. Secondly, I didn't want to burden others with my troubles. Most of them didn't want to know how hard it was because they wouldn't know what to say other than "I am sorry." To make it easier on them, I gave them an easy out by not having the conversation.

   I was sure doctors, lawyers, talk show hosts, firemen, and even the president of the United States had no clue what loneliness as a caregiver felt like. I knew *lonely* was lying to me, but I couldn't prove otherwise.

   I moved on. I was looking for this beautiful grasp of sunshine called *joy*. I vaguely remembered this feeling. Maybe it was from my childhood? I had so many bad feelings now that I couldn't remember what good feelings were or what they felt like.

   I know joy existed. I read about it in every self-help book. I was begging for joy to appear in the box but to no avail. It was nowhere to be found. *Please, joy, reveal yourself.* I wanted to know what *joy* felt like so badly I burst into tears as I scrounged through the feelings box.

I finally realized someone had stolen joy from my feelings box. That wasn't fair. Who could I report this theft to? This was a crime against humanity. Was there a feelings enforcement division at my local police department? Maybe it was a federal agency?

Chapter 18

*S*teve had MSA for at least six years. The level of caregiving he required was significant and only increasing. After years of piecing together a care team of Joanne for a couple of hours in the morning, his mom in the afternoon, and the kids, we prayed for the right person to help while I was at work. For us, me quitting just wasn't a financial option. Joy, a friend from church, was the angel that stepped in. She took on the task of caregiving full time during the day, so Steve could have consistent care and help while I was at work.

Joy was our age, and our families had been friends for several years. She wasn't a trained nurse but learned to do everything needed to care for him. She became Steve's lifeline during the day and my support. She knew Steve loved visits to the grocery store and would regularly load him up in the van and drive him to the grocery store. This accomplished our grocery shopping, gave Steve a chance to go out on an adventure, and helped save my sanity. He did well for about five months, and then MSA reminded us who was the boss of our lives.

One night in mid-spring, Steve tugged on me in the middle of the night to let me know he had to get up to go to the bathroom. How I wished we didn't have to go through this on a regular basis; however, he would never succumb to adult diapers. He wanted me to get him up to the toilet and use the self-catheter. We tried to avoid using a foley catheter long-term, as Steve was prone to persistent UTIs. He was concerned the foley catheter would make him more susceptible. As I tried to get him transferred out of bed into the wheelchair, he was weaker than usual and fell to the floor. Usually, between the two of us, we could get him back up and into the bed. He could lock his arms and I pulled.

Tonight, was different, and I couldn't get him to move at all. Within a few short minutes, he started having trouble catching his breath. Realizing he was in trouble; I called the ambulance to take him to the emergency room. It was the first time I had to call an ambulance in our entire marriage, but I knew I couldn't get him in the van to take him to the ER, and he needed help soon.

He ended up in the worst shape he had ever been and was quickly placed in the ICU. Steve could not communicate with the hospital staff other than to blink his eyes or somewhat move his head in a yes or no, so they relied on me to interpret what he might need and provide guidance on his condition.

His doctor told me his oxygen levels were low and prepared me for the reality that he may never leave the hospital alive. It turned out he had aspiration pneumonia. He spent five days in the ICU and several more in a regular hospital room as he recovered enough to go home. He survived the ICU stay but came home bedridden.

During this time, several of Steve's doctors suggested that he consider hospice again. For at least two years before

Chapter 18

this, his doctors had recommended that Steve consider hospice or a nursing care facility because of the level of daily care he required. At this point, he wasn't even strong enough to sit up in the wheelchair. He was unable to eat, swallowing was difficult at best, and breathing was labored, to where he often would struggle to take in a breath. MSA slowly destroys the organs in your autonomic nervous system. If your body does something automatically without thought, like swallowing and breathing, it is fair game for MSA.

During our last visit to the Mayo Clinic, his doctors had advised us that during the final stages of the disease, it is often respiratory failure that patients succumb to. He was now experiencing a higher level of respiratory failure.

Steve refused to hear of hospice. To him, hospice meant giving up. I didn't see it as giving up; I saw it as someone to help guide us through decisions and potentially offer me some respite from caregiving, but it wasn't going to happen.

Though he could no longer go to the Mayo Clinic or make a visit to his doctor for care, he refused hospice. While it was his decision ultimately, I was unhappy about the decision as I was exhausted beyond imagination. I felt I had no choice but to put resentment out of my mind and respect his decision.

He came home a few days before my birthday. Caregiving had consumed so many birthdays I didn't want to celebrate this one.

No worries, Kim took care of it for me. She surprised me with a pedicure and then offered to follow me back to my house. Unbeknownst to me, she had planned a surprise party at my house with my friend Tammy and another friend named Kim.

It was the best birthday I had in more than ten years, even though Steve was confined to the hospital bed. Kim helped me open the back door to the porch, and we wheeled Steve's hospital bed on the back porch to enjoy the fresh air and birthday cake. I still smile when I think about it. I think I completely gave in at this point. I was so thankful to have a friend willing to do this for me. She genuinely just wanted to be my friend; no ulterior motive, and she really did have a heart of gold.

Shortly after my birthday and the return home from the hospital, a home health nurse came out to do an assessment. Because Steve was a disabled veteran and now bedridden, he qualified for a special VA program, where a doctor would periodically make a home visit. The next day, a doctor came to visit Steve and quickly assessed the severity of the situation and his condition. The doctor asked Steve one question, "The next time your breathing becomes compromised, and it will happen again, do you want to go through what you just went through in the hospital?" Steve despised being in the hospital; every time he went and had to stay, his muscles would atrophy even more from laying in the bed, and he would lose more of the tiny amount of strength and independence he had. He simply said, "No." I said nothing. I wanted this to be his decision alone, and I would support whatever decision he made. He, and he alone, decided to enter hospice. I was eternally grateful to that doctor for recognizing the toll hospital visits were taking on Steve and the increasing level of caregiving was taking on me.

Chapter 19

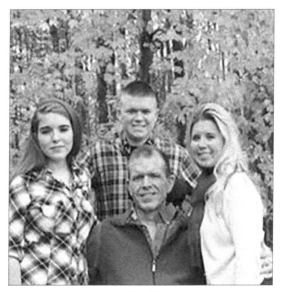

Our family

It was a Thursday night nearly six years into Steve's MSA. I was driving home from work, and I was exhausted. Of course, I was always exhausted, but on this night, little sleep and no free time hit harder, and I was worried about how I would manage to put on my caregiver hat when I walked in the door. How could anyone be a good caregiver in this situation?

At this point, Steve was confined to the hospital bed. It was very difficult to get him in the wheelchair and transfer him. Over the last five weeks since he had come home from the hospital, he had developed a large, deep pressure sore on his backside that required daily wound care. A wound care nurse visited three times a week to change the dressings and check on it. The rest of the time, Joy, our friend and his daytime caregiver, changed the dressings during the day, and I at night and on weekends.

I was now working from home when I could to help manage hospice care and would go to the office the rest of the week. Those days at the office were a welcome escape from the medical world I lived in at home. Work gave me an opportunity to have adult conversations and solve problems that didn't involve medical terminology, catheters, and MSA.

Usually, my hour-long drive home from work was a bit of *me* time, my only time alone, and not caring for any other human being. Often, I called my family or friends. Tonight, I didn't want to talk to anyone. I needed every bit of my being to pray. Since I was driving, praying with my eyes closed and head bowed was out of the question. My prayers tonight were out loud to God.

I regularly prayed multiple times a day. Tonight's prayer was raw and deeply emotional. Tonight, after six years of caregiving, I admitted defeat to this cruel disease. I don't know why tonight was any different. I just felt depleted with little left to give of myself. I was too exhausted to want to do anything but close my eyes and drift off into a deep, long sleep.

Chapter 19

Driving on autopilot, I cried out to God in the most honest, deep, gut-wrenching way I had ever done. I said to God, "I don't know what the future holds. I don't know how much longer You will ask me to be a caregiver, but I am going to be honest, God. I don't want to do this any longer. I am so tired. I need rest. However, I have complete trust in You, and if You determine that I need to be a caregiver for two more years, I will do it for two more years. I won't give up. I am just being honest with You when I tell You I don't want to do it. Please forgive me." Wow, that was the first time I had been completely honest with God about what I was feeling. Up until then, I had just thanked Him in my prayers for giving me strength to keep going.

When I got home, Hailey, a young family friend who had recently started helping with Steve's care for a couple of hours in the afternoon so that Joy didn't have to work so many hours, had made chicken nuggets for Steve. A little strange, I thought, to fix him chicken nuggets since he had a feeding tube and could barely swallow anything, but he had indicated to her that he would like them by pointing out letters on his Styrofoam board with the alphabet on it; a kind of makeshift typewriter. At this point, I rarely questioned crazy decisions like this. How do you tell a dying man he can't have chicken nuggets?

I got Steve ready for bed about 10:00 p.m. He now slept in the hospital bed in the living room. I had been sleeping on the couch so I could be in the same room with him in case he needed me. That night, he told me he wanted to sleep in our bed by pointing at our bedroom and sort of shaking his head no when I tried to get his bed ready. Unhappy to hear this, I tried to talk him out of it. Moving him into our bed was a chore. The hospital bed was easier on my back and safer on him. In our bed, I would have to move him and position pillows in all sorts of contortions to keep him safe and comfortable.

    I was too tired to argue, so we moved into our bedroom. About 12:30 a.m., Steve started shivering. He didn't seem cold; it was the strangest type of shivering. To me, he seemed scared. I wrapped my arms around him as tightly as I could and swaddled him, rocking him a little bit, and saying, "It's okay. It's okay." Soon we both fell back asleep.

    Friday, I woke up with anticipation because Emily would be graduating from high school the next day. This day was important for Steve too. When he first learned that he had MSA six years ago, he told me he wanted to do everything he could to live to see Emily's high school graduation. I was going to be working from home and taking off early to get things ready for Emily's graduation party from high school. For the first time in a couple of years, we had an exciting weekend planned. We were having a family get-together at our house. All our family, friends from church, and some of Emily's friends from school would be coming over. We were all excited to have something to look forward to other than our usual weekends spent restocking medicine.

    We had company coming too. Steve's best friend Mike, who he had served with on the USS John F Kennedy and was now living near Seattle, Washing, was coming to Tennessee to see him. He had not seen or talked to Mike in years. Mike just happened to be making a trip to visit

Chapter 19

other family in the south and wanted to stop in and see Steve while he was this way. It worked out great because he would be here for Emily's graduation as well. For the first time in a long time, I was excited because we would have company.

Mike had stayed close with Steve. After Steve could no longer communicate, Mike would call or text me to check on Steve. Mike told me he would be driving in from visiting another family member in South Carolina that Friday and would probably be at our house around noon.

Friday morning, I woke up around 6:30 a.m. Steve was still asleep. Rarely did Steve sleep later than me. With him waking up last night, I figured he was tired. I quietly slipped out of bed so I didn't wake up Steve. I went into the spare bathroom and threw on a pair of jeans and a V-neck pink cotton shirt.

Once dressed, I went into the kitchen to make my breakfast tea and catch up on the news. I kept checking on Steve, but he seemed to be sleeping peacefully. About 8:00 a.m., Joy showed up to help take care of Steve during the day. When she walked into the bedroom, I put my finger to my mouth to motion quiet and whispered to her to prepare his medicine as he was still sleeping. With Steve still asleep, Joy had a few minutes head-start to the day. Kim and I had made plans to go shopping later that afternoon and get the cake for Emily's graduation party.

Dr. Jayne, Steve's doctor from hospice, was due to come by the house to evaluate him at 10:00 a.m. She had admitted him into hospice about a month ago and wanted to see how he was doing.

By 9:30 a.m., Steve still hadn't awoken. Both Joy and I were now concerned as he was usually up by this time. He was breathing and seemed to be okay. He just wasn't waking up.

By 9:45, I became very concerned. Finally, I heard Dr. Jayne's car pulling into the driveway. I flew out to her car and blurted, "Come quickly to the house. I think something is wrong with Steve. He isn't waking up."

She grabbed her stethoscope and rushed into the house. In the few seconds that I was outside with her, his breathing had become fast, with short breaths.

Dr. Jayne quickly leaned over the bed and listened to Steve's breathing. "We need to get his breathing under control," she said. "Call the hospice nurse on duty and tell her you need morphine immediately, or he is going to die."

I was in shock. A short time ago, I had been having tea and watching the news, and now Dr. Jayne was telling me Steve might die.

I felt almost paralyzed and was so thankful Joy was there to help me think. I called the hospice nurse to bring the morphine. While I was waiting on the nurse to show up, I called Kim to tell her what was happening and let her know I probably couldn't go shopping that afternoon to get things for Emily's graduation party. What Dr. Jayne told me had not sunk in.

Kim was at the house within a half-hour with an overnight bag in tow. She had been through this with other family members and knew what I was in for. I was clueless, numb, in a trance, and unable to absorb the words Dr. Jayne was saying.

Chapter 19

After the hospice nurse arrived, administered the morphine, and assessed Steve, they came to talk to me.

Holding my hand, Dr. Jayne and the hospice nurse looked into my eyes and said, quietly. "Steve won't last through the night. You need to call family and friends to give them the chance to say goodbye."

What? I was in complete shock. *Last night he was asking for chicken nuggets on his Styrofoam makeshift keyboard, and today you are telling me out of the blue he is going to die.*

What was she talking about?

Thankfully, Kim and Joy were there to listen to the instructions. Dr. Jayne said Steve might make it a few hours or a few days. There was no way to know for certain. They gave specific instructions for administering the morphine and things to watch for. I remained in a trance, unable to process what they were saying. It was like they were speaking a foreign language to me.

Kim and Joy helped me make phone calls to all the immediate family. In the middle of making phone calls, I realized Steve's friend Mike was on his way here. Yesterday I talked to him and told him how excited we were to see him, and today Steve might die.

He was close to the house when Kim called him, so I told her to tell him to come on. I asked Mike to stay with us and spend time with Steve. Mike had not seen Steve in five years, and now he was walking in on what was likely Steve's very last day on earth. We cleared the trapeze over the bed, extra medical supplies, and equipment out of the bedroom and brought in chairs for family to sit. I crawled into bed next to him and sat there all day.

Steve's mom and his brother Mike came to the house and sat with him all day amidst their own grief and pain. As more family and close friends came in, we talked, sang hymns, laughed about memories, and cried. Around 8:00 p.m., Steve's breathing seemed to improve slightly, and most of the family went home to get rest. I was convinced this meant tomorrow he would wake up, and this would all be a bad dream.

Kim suggested this would be a good time for me to be alone with Steve. I shut the bedroom door and curled up next to him to just talk. I didn't know what to say, but I believed he could hear me. I had seen this in movies before where loved ones say their last goodbyes. I told him I loved him. I didn't say goodbye; I couldn't bear it. I had this terrible fear he would wake up the next morning and ask me why I would say goodbye to him as if he were dying. I still thought he might make it through this and not die.

Around 10:00 p.m., his breathing changed again and became more labored and shallower. Kim called all the close family and suggested they come back. She didn't think he would make it through the night. I thought she was crazy. The Steve I knew was going to wake up Saturday morning and ask for scrambled eggs for breakfast.

At 11:00 p.m., Emily came in and offered to sing a song. This was unusual because Emily had never sung in front of anyone, even though she had a beautiful voice. She sang to Steve an acapella version of "If We are Honest" by Francesca Battistelli. It was the most beautiful song I had ever heard. There were fifteen people in the room. Jacob, Emily, and I held Steve's hand.

Chapter 19

At 12:20 a.m., the last of our family members went home. Everyone was exhausted. Most had been at the house since early afternoon. Jacob and Emily went back to bed.

None of us were crying at this point because we were physically and emotionally exhausted. I think Jacob and Emily understood what was happening, but I couldn't speak of it. How could I tell them that Dad might not wake up in the morning? I had this fear that if I spoke the words that he would die, I couldn't take them back. Naively, I wanted to believe that if I thought he would wake up on Saturday morning, he *would* wake up. I was numb, exhausted, terrified, and yet holding onto any hope of him improving all at the same time. Kim and my friend Rachel, who had been there all day, offered to sit in the bedroom and keep watch on things so I could go to sleep.

I put on my pajamas and crawled under the covers next to Steve. I tried to go to sleep but was too on edge because of something Kim had said to me earlier in the evening. "Once all the family leaves, it won't be long before Steve passes." She later told me she had been at the bedside of her grandparents when they had passed. *How could she know? The doctors didn't know when.*

I looked at the clock. It was 12:41 a.m., twenty minutes after the last family member left and ten minutes after we turned off the light. I got into bed, and the house finally seemed quiet after all the family coming and going throughout the day. Steve seemed to be about the same, and then, without warning, drew in one last gasp of air and never exhaled.

I held my breath as I waited for him to exhale. He never did.

I went from being a full-time exhausted caregiver to alone: alone, empty, lost, grieving. My entire world changed in one last breath. I immediately realized Steve had accomplished exactly what he had set out to do once he learned he had MSA. He had made it to Emily's high school graduation. He died Saturday morning at 12:41 a.m., and Emily was supposed to graduate high school at 9:00 a.m.

The Saturday night we renewed our vows in our country church were coming to mind now. "In sickness and health, till death do us part," I had said, "I do." I never anticipated what that really meant. I never anticipated that the church where we renewed our vows would be where we would bury Steve, and our hopes and dreams as a couple would be gone just six years later. Had I done everything I could have done as his wife and caregiver? I felt like I had, but MSA didn't care. It took Steve anyway.

In that one last breath, I felt so many emotions. Heartbreak in losing my husband of twenty-eight years, sadness in what that meant to my life, Jacob and Emily having lost their dad, and anger in how much of our lives had been taken by this disease. Still, something in me recognized the beauty in death. God had allowed me the opportunity to be present during the very last breath my husband took on this earth. This was a gift. I had been entrusted with one of the most sacred experiences anyone could ever have.

Conclusion

The first thirty days after Steve died were the most difficult. Immersed in a whirlwind of emotions, I felt completely lost and alone. I couldn't even make easy decisions. During Steve's funeral, I wanted to display near the casket at the funeral home one of Steve's Mediterranean cruise jackets from the navy. The funeral home director asked me if I would like a wooden or metal hanger to hang the jacket on. My mind went blank, my body numb. I looked at Kim and asked her what to do. "The wooden hanger," she said, knowing my mind was too muddled to think. It would be one of many decisions she helped me make.

I tried to go back to work a week after Steve died. I stayed for a few hours but realized I couldn't focus enough to make any decisions. I felt useless.

Unfortunately, I had already used all my FMLA throughout the year to care for Steve, and I had no vacation or sick time life. Still, I went to my boss and asked for thirty days off. Compassionate, he understood I was going through an extremely difficult time. He allowed me to take thirty days off unpaid.

At this point, I didn't care if I was paid or not. I couldn't do my job effectively, so being there was pointless. I felt like I had nothing left to give anyone. Having used all my energy and resources on caregiving for the last six years, I was empty.

The time off helped me navigate all the strong emotions going through me. My days were a roller coaster. I went from bursts of energy to being unable to do anything. I wasn't even sure what to do now. For the last six years, I didn't have free time. As a new widow, I didn't even know if it was appropriate to enjoy my free time or sit at home and sulk. Deep down, I was relieved not to be a caregiver anymore, but it didn't feel appropriate because it meant I had to lose Steve to lose caregiving.

A couple of weeks after Steve died, Kim showed up one sunny day in her Jeep with the top off and asked if I wanted to go for a ride. For me, the idea was foreign. Never in my past six years did I have the liberty to just hop in a Jeep and go for a ride.

With the sun on us, the wind in my hair, and a glorious feeling of freedom, we rode to the Hiwassee River. It was a beautiful river about thirty minutes away from my house, but I had never been to it. Kim went regularly. She kayaked there and her, husband Riley liked to fish there. Everyone we passed seemed relaxed as if they didn't have a care in the world. I felt like a teenager on summer vacation, filled with happiness I hadn't felt in years. Feeling free and happy filled me with guilt. *How could you?* I thought to myself. *Steve had just died!*

People tell you it will take a year or so for things to get back to normal and stabilize and not to make any big

Conclusion

decisions the first year. In retrospect, I now understand the wisdom of this. If there was a book on *How to Be a Widow for Dummies*, I didn't find it. Every day was a new challenge, and a lot of people have different opinions on what is proper behavior.

I changed much that first year. I went from being a wife and caregiver to a widow at forty-eight years old. That was a lot to process. I went from being physically worn down, emotionally drained, constantly grieving, and tired to a period of growth. I went from holding onto death to learning a new life.

Almost a year after Steve had died, a friend of mine, Jeff, who runs an investment company, asked me to speak at the annual Valentine's Day widow's luncheon they held. He wanted me to share my story of Steve's illness, caregiving, and how our faith had strengthened us.

After making a mental outline of what I wanted to cover, I got up to speak to about thirty people. They were all different ages but mostly older widows and widowers. As I was talking, I realized something I hadn't yet figured out: *I* was one of the widows in this group. This realization made my life and everything we had been through starkly real.

When I finished, several people came up to me and thanked me for sharing the brutal honesty about what it was like to be a caregiver. It wasn't always nice. Sometimes I was mad at my situation, sometimes I was tired and cranky, and sometimes I wanted to run away.

Driving home, I thought about how every time I came to an obstacle, and I thought I couldn't go on, when I had no energy left for another step, no patience, no desire, and no strength, I would say out loud, *I have no patience, no desire, and no strength.* It was negative, defeating, and victim-playing. Still, something in me crazily hoped that saying the words out loud or whispering them if anyone was in earshot might give me the push, I needed to move forward to have the energy to be a caregiver for one more day.

Rare individuals like Mother Teresa had the strength to sustain years of being a caregiver without a break. I wasn't a saint. I would mumble under my breath sometimes about how much I hated my life, too ashamed to admit to anyone how I was feeling, too weak to do what was necessary to do.

In writing this book, I realize I had more strength than I imagined existed within me. Six years of progressively intensifying caregiving while working full time, spending two hours commuting to work, and being both Mom and Dad to our two teenagers was unimaginably difficult. Yet I did it. I *was* strong, even though I didn't often recognize my strength and resilience; hope was elusive, but I never gave up. Occasionally, I stopped in the journey and collapsed into tears, but then I got myself up and plugged on.

Despite everything and through it all, I felt blessed. God never forgot about what I was going through. He always sent me help, some person to encourage me, someone to secretly bring me dinner, a text to brighten my day, and a good day with Emily and Jacob. I knew someday I would have to share what I went through with other caregivers. I wanted to give them hope and share some strategies.

Conclusion

God had a plan at work, and He was gracious enough to let me join in. I had connected with a lot of people through social media, friends, and church who contacted me to ask how I kept up the pace. Generally, my answer was something along the lines of "God is better to me than I deserve and gives me the strength."

For a Christian, it's easier to understand because you derive your entire being, your center of life, from His strength. Without God, you can survive, but hope will be elusive. If you are a caregiver at this very moment, it may not feel like it, but you will survive. I have learned that God does not waste any amount of heartache, pain, or struggle you are going through.

With the right perspective, you will not only survive but also learn to embrace your current situation as an opportunity to grow.

Acknowledgments

Writing this book has been a journey of heartache and hope. The story isn't mine alone. God allowed me to become a caregiver to teach me and to strengthen me. I am eternally grateful for Steve's and every veterans service to our country. Steve's faith and courage taught me so much throughout this journey as his wife and caregiver. Jacob and Emily, I love more than they can imagine. This journey has been so difficult on both of them, and I am extremely proud of the way they have matured despite the trauma and grief they have been through.

There were so many people along the last six years who have encouraged me to write this book. My best friend and soulmate of a sister, Kim, daily encouraged me, sat in the bedroom with me as Steve passed away, and adopted my whole family into her family. She and I both have a heart for caregivers. She continues to lift me up and together we pray for those of you facing similar situations as you read this book. My acknowledgments will never come close to what she means to me.

Our church family at Rogers Creek Baptist Church in Athens, Tennessee. The pastor at the time, Jeff, and his wife Rachel became close friends of ours. Jeff mentored Steve and visited with him as a friend. Rachel cooked and cared for the whole family. She called me every day on my way to work to let me vent, read books to me, and prayed with me as I drove. Their tremendous love and support helped us survive.

Dwight and Donna, whom I can only describe as two of the most thoughtful, loving people I have ever met. They have done many things behind the scenes to help us throughout the years. They have been close friends, but I love them like family.

Steve's brother Mike, who became a brother to me in turn. I love you, Mike and I am so appreciative of everything you have done to be there for us. My niece Alisha, for the continued encouragement to write the book.

My mother-in-law Louise. She daily cared for Steve while I was at work and has opened her heart to me as a daughter.

One of my longest friendships and an amazing voice of reason continues to be Tammy. We rarely got to see each other during the six years Steve was sick since she lives in another state, however our daily phone calls gave me the encouragement to keep going and as a Certified Registered Nurse Anesthetist, she had the knowledge to help me decipher some of the medical terminologies. Thank you for always helping me see the other side of things, encouraging me, and loving me through it all.

Travis, whom I met after starting this book is one of the most thoughtful, loving, and caring men God could have blessed me with. He is a light in my life and I love him tremendously. He has supported me constantly,

Acknowledgments

encouraged me, and has loved my entire family including Steve's family, as if they were his own.

Steve's cousin Tommy and his whole family, showed up every single time I called. He regularly came over to check on Steve, spend time with him, and help with anything we needed.

My entire family in Ohio, but especially my sister Michelle. She is the glue that holds our whole family together and daily called me just to check on me. My mom; my sister Melenie; my dad, who recently passed away; my cousin Paul; my close friend Cheryl, and my Aunt Barbara. I love you all.

A very special friend and Steve's caregiver, Joy. Joy cared for Steve about the last eight months of his life. Her ability to take on such a tremendous task and make Steve's last month's happy with grocery store trips and helping him order candy from Amazon were blessings.

Connie a delightful lady and truly compassionate friend we met through church. More than once she drove six plus hours from Illinois to check on Steve.

My credit union family, with special friends in Tennessee including Dale and her husband Dewayne, Kathy, Kim, Barbara, Shelli, Jamin, Melissa, Virginia, and Lisa. My credit union compliance family from around the country, especially Donna, Kristen, Gaye, Renee, Bill, Charlotte, Mike, Richard, and Donya. Your lifelong friendship, love, and concern mean the world to me to this day.

Inheritance of Hope. This small, life-changing organization has a mission to inspire hope in young families with a parent with a terminal illness. They rescued our family during our darkest hour and provided us with the love and support on our only family vacation we were able to take during his entire illness. I have since gone on to pay this love forward and volunteer to help other families. I encourage you to learn more about them at www.inheritanceofhope.org.

The Defeat MSA Alliance. Realizing that much of the current attention is focused on more widely known diseases, Multiple System Atrophy is often overlooked. MSA patients are confronted with a dim prognosis and left with few options. Staffed entirely by volunteers the Defeat MSA Alliance aspires to balance efforts to support patients, educate medical professionals, raise public awareness, nurture promising research and advocate for the MSA community. Learn more at www.defeatmsa.org.

Finally, I want to acknowledge every caregiver who is taking his/her valuable time to read this story. I am not sure where you are in your journey right now, but please know wherever it is, there is hope. It may not seem like it, but your journey is temporary. Caregiving is often a thankless and unseen job, but you are one of the most valuable persons in the lives of your loved ones.

CPSIA information can be obtained
at www.ICGtesting.com
Printed in the USA
BVHW081216160223
658645BV00001B/204